WORKBOOK

MATERNAL NEWBORN NURSING CARE

The Nurse, the Family, and the Community

FOURTH EDITION

Marcia L. London, RNC, MSN, NNP
Associate Professor and Director
Neonatal Nurse Practitioner Program
Beth-El College of Nursing
Colorado Springs, Colorado

Patricia Wieland Ladewig, RNC, PhD
Professor and Dean
School for Health Care Professions
Regis University
Denver, Colorado

Sally B. Olds, RNC, MS
Associate Professor
Beth-El College of Nursing
Colorado Springs, Colorado

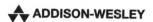 **ADDISON-WESLEY**

An imprint of Addison Wesley Longman, Inc.

Menlo Park, California • Reading, Massachusetts • New York • Harlow, England
Don Mills, Ontario • Sydney • Mexico City • Madrid • Amsterdam

We dedicate this book to our families—with love.
David, Craig, and Matthew London
Tim, Ryan, and Erik Ladewig
Joe, Scott, and Allison Olds

Executive Editor: Patricia L. Cleary
Project Editor: Virginia Simione Jutson
Managing Editor: Wendy Earl
Production Editor: David Novak
Composition: The Left Coast Group, Inc.
Cover Designer: Yvo Riezebos Design

ISBN 0-8053-5628-2
1 2 3 4 5 6 7 8 9 10—VG—01 00 99 98 97

Addison Wesley Longman, Inc.
2725 Sand Hill Road
Menlo Park, California 94025

Preface

Maternal-newborn nurses are responsible for a complex, highly specialized body of knowledge related to the needs of the child-bearing family, whether normal or at-risk. In recent years, that knowledge has expanded rapidly, as have the technology and complex ethical issues surrounding pregnancy and birth. In addition, these issues must be taught in a shorter period of time.

The *Maternal-Newborn Nursing Workbook* can assist in that effort by providing a concise, up-to-date review of essential maternal-newborn nursing theoretical content emphasizing application of the nursing process and critical thinking in clinical maternity settings. Selected women's health issues are also explored.

All major maternity texts include content related to the human reproductive system and to the antepartal, intrapartal, postpartal, and neonatal periods, although their sequences may vary. This workbook can also be used with most of the major maternity nursing texts, no matter what their organization. It is specifically designed to be used with *Ladewig, London, and Olds: Maternal-Newborn Nursing: The Nurse, the Family, and the Community*, Fourth Edition. The subjects follow the same sequence as in the textbook, although a few textbook chapters may be combined into one workbook chapter. To assist the student, we have identified the pertinent corresponding text chapters at the beginning of each workbook chapter. The workbook is appropriate for all types of nursing programs—baccalaureate, associate degree, and diploma. Nurses involved in refresher courses or just entering this specialty area will also find it helpful. Practicing nurses may find it helpful, too, especially in assessment and critical clinical decision-making.

Features New to This Edition

This workbook emphasizes the application and synthesis of an expanding research-based, maternal newborn nursing clinical knowledge. Since we learn best through active learning, we have provided critical thinking scenarios to further develop your critical decision-making and prioritizing skills. *Critical thinking challenge situations* are presented and the student is asked to prioritize nursing actions. *Critical thinking in practice sequences* have been developed for selected normal and complication chapters to provide realistic clinical practice situations. Clinical data is presented and the student is guided through the decision-making process for a particular situation.

Because we believe that sound clinical judgment develops from theoretical knowledge, research, and practical experience, most of the items in this workbook are based on clinical situations. Recognizing the rich cultural heritage of our diverse population, many of these client situations include ethnic families.

Working with the childbearing family is an intensely rewarding interactive nursing experience. The review of these clinical experiences and/or a personal childbearing experience increases our understanding of the universal childbirth/parenting experience. We have provided the student with opportunities in the *Reflections* feature to revisit and ponder those experiences.

Some of the questions are related to factual material, and students can verify their answers easily in the provided answer section at the end of the workbook. However, for those questions that require synthesis and more application, we have established a critical thinking dialogue with the student to assist in self-assessment. In addition we have provided the pertinent pages in the textbook for the student for those more complex questions.

Clarification of Terms

Although we recognize that the men in nursing are becoming more involved in the provision of maternity care, women are still the major care providers. Therefore, whenever possible, we have avoided sexist pronouns in referring to the nurse. When this was not possible, we have used the female pronoun.

By the same token, we appreciate the fact that the individual who is most significant to the pregnant woman may be her husband, the father of the child, another family member, or simply a good friend, male or female. Thus we have provided both traditional "husband-wife" situations, and situations involving other support persons.

Acknowledgments

First, we would like to recognize the students who reviewed the previous edition of this workbook. They approached their review seriously and provided many candid comments. They identified material that they felt was unclear and added valuable suggestions that enhance this edition.

We thank the nurse educators and practicing nurses who reviewed this material and offered their suggestions and comments. Their input helped us focus on the most pertinent material and offered a broader perspective.

Last but not least, we thank our families. We recognize the countless ways that they continue to help us and the sacrifices that they make as we pursue this other love. Women can accomplish any goal, however, combining marriage, family, intellectual challenges and a career requires a supportive, adaptive, responsive family. Each of us is blessed with such a family. We love them.

M.L.L.
P.W.L.
S.B.O.

Contents

1 | Contemporary Maternal Newborn Care

This chapter corresponds to Chapter 1 in the 4th edition of *Maternal-Newborn Nursing Care: The Nurse, the Family, and the Community.*

Roles and Standards

1. Maternity nurses function in a variety of roles in providing care to childbearing families. Define each of the following roles with emphasis on educational background and scope of function:

   a. Certified registered nurse (RNC) — Takes National certification Exam

   b. Clinical nurse specialist (CNS) — Has a master's degree and speccalized knowledge and competence in a specific clinical area.

   c. Nurse practitioner (NP) — Received specialized education in a masters degree program or a certificate program and can function in an advance practice role

   PS see functions

   d. Certified nurse-midwife (CNM) Educated in the two disciplines of nursing and midwifery. Certified by the American College of Nurse-Midwives

2. Which of the following would be most qualified to provide prenatal, intrapartal, postpartal, and newborn care for the low-risk childbearing woman?

   a. Acute-care clinical nurse specialist

   b. Certified nurse-midwife

   c. Lay midwife

   d. Obstetric or women's health care nurse practitioner

3. Discuss the standards of care that shape maternal-newborn nursing.

p8

Caregivers must respect the pregnant woman's autonomy. The procedure involve health risks to the woman and she retains the right to refuse any surgical procedure.

Descriptive Statistics

4. Define the following terms:

 a. Birth rate — Number of Live births per (1000) people

 b. Infant mortality rate — Number of deaths of infants under 1 year of age per (1000) Live births in a given _population_.

 c. Neonatal mortality — Number of deaths of infants less than 28 days of age per (1000) Live births

 d. Maternal mortality — Number of deaths from any cause during the pregnancy cycle including 42 day postpartal period per (100,000) Live births

5. Identify factors that may contribute to the decrease in the maternal mortality rate.

p13

① Increase use of Hospitals

② Specialized health care personnel by maternity clients

③ Establishment of care centers for high risk mothers and infants

④ Prevent and control of infection with ABT + improved transfusion techniques. The availability of blood + blood products for

6. Perinatal mortality is a combination of

 a. infant death rate and neonatal mortality.

 b. fetal death rate and infant death rate.

 c. neonatal mortality and postneonatal mortality.

 d. fetal death rate and neonatal mortality.

Reflections

There are many difficult ethical issues affecting the childbearing woman and family today. What do you think the most difficult issue will be for you in your maternal-newborn nursing course?

_____

_____

_____

_____

_____

_____

7.   Summarize the primary purposes of the Human Genome Project.

2 | The Reproductive System

This chapter corresponds to Chapter 2 in the 4th edition of *Maternal-Newborn Nursing Care: The Nurse, the Family, and the Community.*

Female Reproductive System

Match the external genitalia structure with its function or characteristics during the childbearing period.

1. _____a_____ Clitoris   a. Produces smegma that has a sexually stimulating odor

2. _____c_____ Labia minora   b. Protects pelvic bones, especially during coitus

3. _____b_____ Mons pubis   c. Rich in sebaceous glands that lubricate and provide bactericidal secretions

4. _____e_____ Paraurethral (Skene's glands)   d. Secretes clear thick mucus that enhances sperm viability and motility

5. _____f_____ Perineal body   e. Secretions lubricate vaginal vestibule to facilitate sexual intercourse

6. _____d_____ Vulvovaginal (Bartholin's glands)   f. Site of episiotomy and lacerations

7. Figure 2–1 on page 5 shows the female internal reproductive organs. Identify the structures that are indicated.

8. Briefly discuss the function(s) of the vagina.

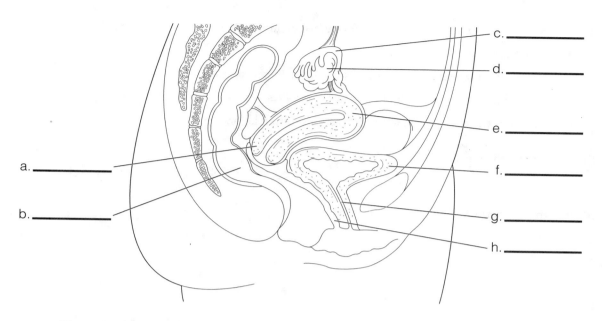

Figure 2–1   Female internal reproductive organs.

9.   What factors can alter the vagina's pH and decrease its self-cleansing action?

10.   Label the uterine structures indicated in Figure 2–2.

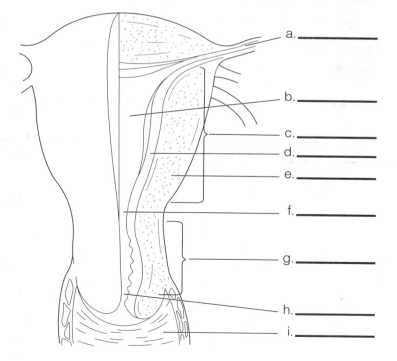

Figure 2–2   Anatomy of the uterus.

11. The figure-eight pattern of the middle layer of uterine muscle fibers

   a. causes cervical effacement.

   b. constricts large uterine blood vessels when the fibers contract.

   c. forms sphincters at fallopian tube attachment sites.

   d. maintains the effects of uterine contractions during labor.

12. Briefly describe the function of the endometrium.

13. Identify three functions of the cervical mucosa.

   a.

   b.

   c.

14. A group of adolescents is waiting for pregnancy tests in a clinic. One of the girls asks about infections. The nurse explains that certain body functions protect the female from infection of the reproductive organs. Which of the following protects the female from infection of the reproductive organs?

   a. Alkaline pH and smegma secreted from the clitoris

   b. Acidic pH and bacteriostatic cervical mucosa

   c. Neutral pH of 7.5 and bactericidal secretions of the labia minora

   d. pH of 4 to 5 and secretions of the Skene's ducts

15. Identify the location and function of each of the following uterine ligaments:

Ligament	Location	Function
Broad ligaments		
Round ligaments		
Cardinal ligaments		

Ligament	Location	Function
Infundibulopelvic ligament		
Uterosacral ligaments		
Ovarian ligaments		

16. What are the primary functions of the fallopian tubes?

17. In relation to the fallopian tubes, what is the purpose or significance of each of the following?

   a. Fimbria

   b. Isthmus

   c. Ampulla

   d. Muscular layer

   e. Nonciliated goblet cells of the mucosa

   f. Tubal cilia

18. Briefly describe the function of the three layers (tunica albuginea, cortex, medulla) of the ovary.

19. What is (are) the primary function(s) of the ovaries?

20. Label the following pelvic bones and supporting ligaments in Figure 2–3.

Sacrum
Left innominate bone
Symphysis pubis
Right sacroiliac joint
Sacroiliac ligament
Sacrospinous ligament
Sacrotuberous ligament
Coccyx

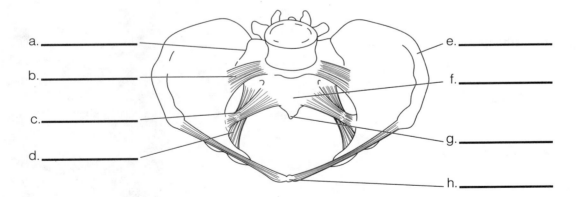

a. _____

b. _____

c. _____

d. _____

e. _____

f. _____

g. _____

h. _____

Figure 2–3 Bony pelvis with ligaments.

21.   Figure 2–4 focuses on the muscles of the pelvic floor. Label the following structures:

Vagina   Ischial tuberosity
Bulbospongiosus muscle   Adductor longus muscle
Gluteus maximus muscle   Pubococcygeus muscle
Ischiocavernosus muscle   External anal sphincter
Iliococcygeus muscle   Urogenital diaphragm

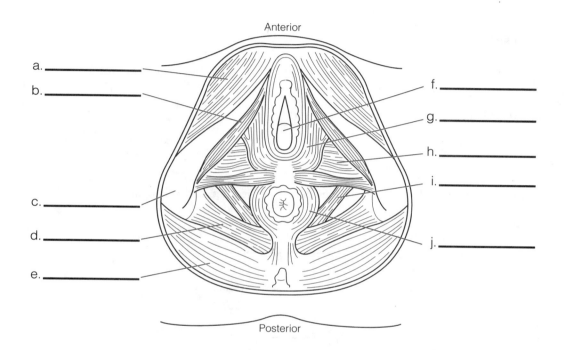

Figure 2–4   Muscles of the pelvic floor.

22.   The major muscle group that forms the pelvic diaphragm is the _____.

23.   Define each of the following terms and briefly identify its implications for childbearing:

   a.   False pelvis

   b.   True pelvis

   c.   Pelvic inlet

   d.   Pelvic outlet

24.   In Figure 2–5, label the false pelvis, true pelvis, pelvic inlet, and pelvic outlet.

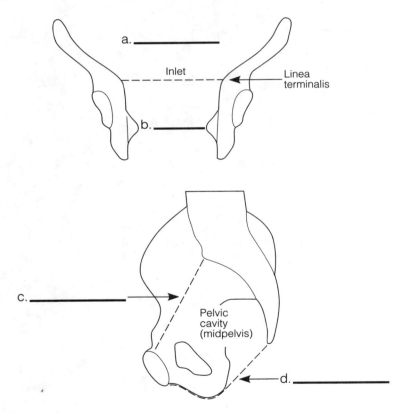

Figure 2–5   Pelvic divisions.

25.   Label the major structures of the breast in Figure 2–6.

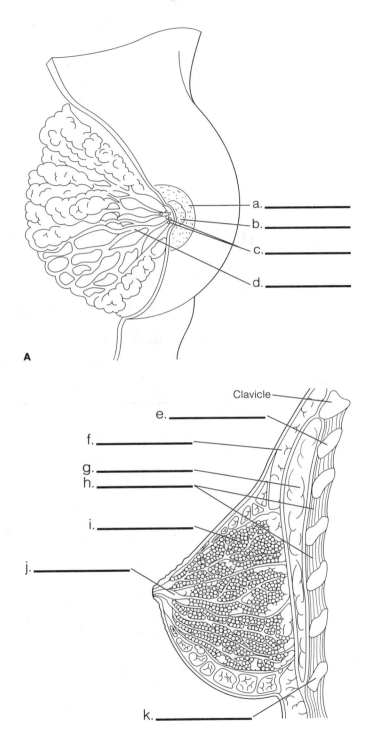

a. _____

b. _____

c. _____

d. _____

A

Clavicle

e. _____

f. _____

g. _____

h. _____

i. _____

j. _____

B

k. _____

Figure 2–6   Anatomy of the breast. **A** Anterior view of partially dissected left breast.
B Sagittal section.

26.   What is the primary function of the tubercles of Montgomery?

27.   What portion of the breast contains the cuboidal epithelial cells that secrete the components of milk?

   a.   Alveoli

   b.   Ducts

   c.   Lactiferous sinuses

   d.   Lobules

Female Reproductive Cycle (FRC)

28.   The female reproductive cycle is made up of two interrelated cycles that occur simultaneously: the

   (a) ————————————— cycle and the (b) ————————————— cycle.

29.   For each of the following hormones involved in ovulation and menstruation, state the source of secretion and the primary function(s).

Hormone	Source	Function(s)
Estrogen		
Progesterone		
Follicle-stimulating hormone (FSH)		
Gonadotropin-releasing hormone (GnRH)		
Luteinizing hormone (LH)		
Prostaglandins (PGE and $PGF_{2\alpha}$)		

30. A girl waiting for a pregnancy test asks the nurse which hormone causes ovulation to occur. The nurse explains that about 18 hours after the peak production of _____, ovulation occurs.

   a. estrogen

   b. FSH (follicle-stimulating hormone)

   c. LH (luteinizing hormone)

   d. progesterone

31. The nurse asks the girl to identify the hormone responsible for enhancing development of the Graafian follicle and rebuilding the endometrium. The right answer would be

   a. estrogen.

   b. FSH–RH (follicle-stimulating hormone–releasing hormone).

   c. GnRH (gonadotropin-releasing hormone).

   d. LHRH (luteinizing hormone–releasing hormone).

32. Describe the process of ovulation and the related changes in the ovarian follicle.

33. Briefly describe the changes that occur in each of the following during the various phases of the menstrual cycle.

   a. Endometrium

   b. Cervical mucosa

34.   Label the following components of the menstrual cycle in Figure 2–7.

Menstrual	Secretory	Follicular	Estrogen
Proliferative	Ischemic	Luteal	Progesterone

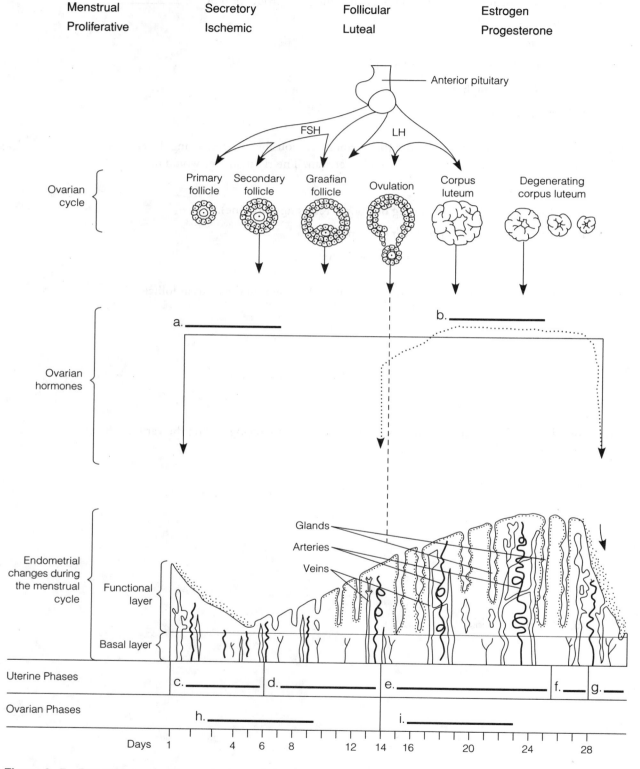

Figure 2–7   Female reproductive cycle: Interrelationships of hormones and the four phases of the uterine cycle and two phases of the ovarian cycle.

Male Reproductive System

35.   The most important purpose for the location of the scrotum is to

    a.   maintain temperature lower than that of the body.

    b.   produce sperm near the point of ejaculation.

    c.   protect the testes and sperm from the effects of the prostate.

    d.   provide room for the convoluted seminiferous tubules.

36.   Complete the following sentences using the words related to the male reproductive structures and functions listed below.

Bulbourethral (Cowper's) glands	penis	seminal vesicles
epididymides	prostate gland	testis
ejaculatory duct	Sertoli cells	testes
Leydig cells	seminal fluid (semen)	vas deferens

The visible male reproductive organs include the (a) _____ and the scrotum. The primary function of the scrotum is protection; it contains the (b) _____,

(c) _____, and (d) _____: the male internal reproductive structures.

Each (e) _____ produces testosterone via the (f) _____, which houses the seminiferous tubules and immature sperm. Maturation of sperm occurs in the

(g) _____, the storage area for mature spermatozoa. Seminiferous tubules contain (h) _____ cells that nourish and protect the spermatocytes. The (i) _____ secretes fluids high in fructose and prostaglandins that nourish sperm and increase their motility. The vas deferens and the duct of a seminal vesicle unite to form a short tube called the (j) _____, which passes through the prostate gland and terminates in the urethra. The (k) _____ gland secretes thin, alkaline fluid containing calcium and other substances that counteract the acidity of ductus and seminal vesicle secretions. The prostate gland secretes substances in the (l) _____. The (m) _____ glands secrete viscous, alkaline fluid rich in mucoproteins, which neutralize the acid in the male urethra and the vagina.

37.   **Memory Check:** Define the following abbreviations.

    a.   FRC   c.   GnRH

    b.   FSH   d.   LH

3 | Conception, Fetal Development, and Special Reproductive Issues

This chapter corresponds to Chapters 3 and 4 in the 4th edition of *Maternal-Newborn Nursing Care: The Nurse, the Family, and the Community*.

Cellular Division

1. Briefly compare mitosis and meiosis.

2. The optimal time for fertilization to occur is (a) _____ hours after ovulation of the ovum and (b) _____ hours after ejaculation.

3. Each sperm and ovum has (a) _____ chromosomes. When sperm and ovum are united, the resulting normal newborn has (b) _____ chromosomes.

4. The (a) _____ chromosome determines the sex of the child. The (b) _____ carries this chromosome.

5. Fertilization occurs in the
   a. cervix.
   b. fallopian tube.
   c. ovary.
   d. uterus.

6. Briefly describe the process of fertilization.

7.   Describe the two processes that the sperm undergoes in order to fertilize the ovum.

   a.

   b.

Cellular Multiplication and Implantation

The zygote continually develops as it travels through the fallopian tube to its site of implantation in the uterus. Match each of the following terms with the appropriate description.

8.   _____ Cleavage   a.   Period of rapid cellular division

9.   _____ Blastomeres   b.   Outer layer of cells that replaces the zona pellucida

10. _____ Morula   c.   Small developing mass of cells held together by zona pellucida

11. _____ Blastocyst   d.   Solid ball of cells

12. _____ Trophoblasts   e.   Inner solid mass of cells after cavity has formed

13. Implantation occurs about (a) _____ to (b) _____ days after fertilization. Briefly describe how implantation occurs.

14. After implantation, the portion of the endometrium that overlies the developing ovum is called
   a.   decidua basalis.
   b.   decidua capsularis.
   c.   decidua luteum.
   d.   decidua vera.

15. The mesoderm germ layer gives rise to the following structures:
   a.   Alimentary canal, lungs, liver, and bladder
   b.   Circulatory system, skin epithelium, and reproductive organs
   c.   Muscles, lungs, and circulatory system
   d.   Nervous system, lungs, and genitourinary system

Embryonic Membranes/Amniotic Fluid

16.   The embryonic membranes begin to form at the time of implantation. Two distinct membranes

develop, the (a) _____ and the (b) _____ .

17.   Describe the normal amount and composition of amniotic fluid.

18.   Using the terms from question 14 and your answers to question 16, fill in the blanks on
Figure 3–1, the early development of the baby.

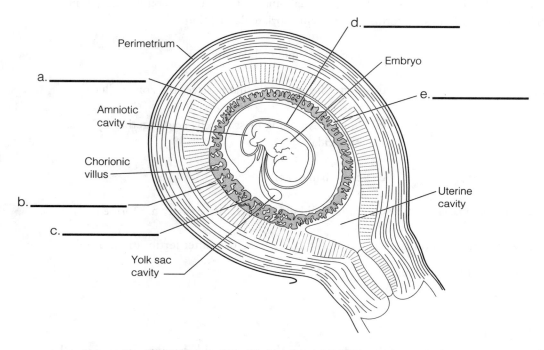

Figure 3–1   Early development of the baby. This figure depicts early development of selected
structures at approximately 8 weeks.

19.   List four functions of amniotic fluid.

a.

b.

c.

d.

Placenta Development and Function

20.   Briefly describe the process through which the placenta and its component structures develop. Also describe the appearance of the maternal and fetal side of the placenta.

21.   Identify three major functions of the placenta.

   a.

   b.

   c.

22.   List the four major placental hormones and their function during pregnancy.

Hormone	Function
a.	
b.	
c.	
d.	

23.   Describe the visual assessments you would want to make of the placenta after birth.

24.   Describe the following stages of human development in utero.

   a.   Embryo

   b.   Fetus

Fetal Circulation

25.   The body stalk, which attaches the embryo to the yolk sac, will develop into the umbilical

   cord. The umbilical cord is made up of (a) _____ vein(s),

   (b) _____ artery(ies), and specialized connective tissue

   called (c) _____, whose function is to (d) _____

   _____.

26.   Circle the answer that correctly completes these sentences.

   The umbilical vein carries (**oxygenated**) or (**deoxygenated**) blood (**to**) or (**away from**)

   the fetus.

   The umbilical arteries carry (**oxygenated**) or (**deoxygenated**) blood (**from**) or (**to**) the

   fetus to the placenta.

27.   Label the following structures in Figure 3–2 and, using arrows, trace the normal pathway of fetal circulation:

Umbilical vein

Foramen ovale

Ductus venosus

Ductus arteriosus

Inferior vena cava

Umbilical arteries

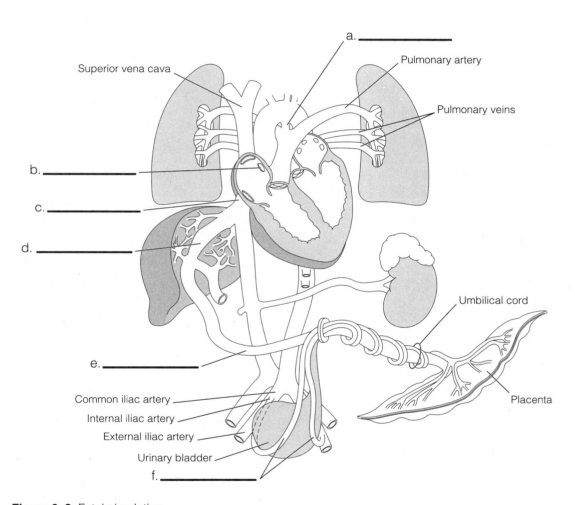

Figure 3–2 Fetal circulation.

28.   Describe the function of each of the following fetal structures during fetal life and the changes that occur after birth.

Fetal	Newborn
a. Umbilical vein	
b. Ductus venosus	
c. Inferior vena cava	
d. Foramen ovale	
e. Ductus arteriosus	
f. Umbilical arteries	

Fetal Development

29. A fetus weighing about 300 gm and measuring 18 cm in length that can actively suck and swallow amniotic fluid is approximately how many weeks' gestation?

    a. 14 weeks

    b. 18 weeks

    c. 20 weeks

    d. 24 weeks

30. You are assisting in a prenatal class on fetal development. Mrs. Elizabeth Oliver, a 22-year-old primigravida, is 14 weeks pregnant and has the following questions. Based on your knowledge of fetal development, how would you respond?

    a. "When will my baby look like a baby?"

    b. "How long is my baby now and how much does it weigh?"

    c. "When will I feel my baby move?"

    d. "When will my baby's heart start beating?"

    e. "When can my baby's sex be identified?"

    f. "Can my baby open its eyes?"

31. Identify four factors that influence embryonic and fetal development.

    a.

    b.

    c.

    d.

Reflections

Feeling movement brings images of the future baby to moms and dads. What have parents told you about this, or what have you personally felt?

_____

_____

_____

_____

_____

_____

_____

_____

_____

_____

_____

32.   The fetus is most vulnerable to congenital malformation development during the first

_____ weeks of life.

Infertility

33.   Define the following terms:

a.   Primary infertility

b.   Secondary infertility

34. During a routine annual examination, your client tells you that she and her husband have been trying to conceive a child for about 8 months but have been unsuccessful. She asks you if there are any actions they can take to increase her chances of getting pregnant. What information would you give her?

35. Describe the correct procedure for taking the BBT and the changes in basal body temperature that will occur throughout a woman's cycle if she is ovulating.

Match the tests below with their correct procedure or purpose.

36. _____ Cervical mucus tests (Ferning, Spinnbarkheit)

    a. Detects changes in cervical mucus due to changing estrogen levels

37. _____ Endometrial biopsy

    b. Examination of uterine cavity and tubes using contrast media instilled through the cervix

38. _____ Postcoital examination (Huhner Test)

    c. Examination of cervical mucus for sperm motility

39. _____ Hysterosalpingography

    d. Examination of uterine lining for secretory changes and receptivity to implantation

40. _____ Gonadotropin levels (LH, FSH assays)

    e. Detects ovulation and corpus luteum function

41. _____ Progesterone assay

    f. Immunological test to determine sperm and cervical mucus compatibility and interaction

42. _____ Sperm immobilization antigen antibody test

    g. Detects follicular development and ovulatory function

43.   Discuss semen analysis as a diagnostic tool in an infertility workup. How is the semen
       collected? What findings indicate a normal semen analysis?

       A sperm count below _____ million/mL indicates probable infertility.

44.   For each of the following medications used to treat infertility, summarize the purpose, method
       of administration, and possible side effects:

       a.   Clomiphene citrate (Clomid Serophene)

       b.   Human menopausal gonadotropin (Pergonal)

       c.   Bromocriptine (Parlodel)

       d.   Gonadotropin-releasing hormone (GnRH)

45. Victor Priolo's father has Huntington's disease and Victor is exhibiting mild symptoms of the disorder. In order to eliminate any possibility of transmitting the disease to their offspring, Victor and his wife, Ann, are considering artificial insemination. An effective procedure would be to use

   a. donor sperm, implanted in Ann.

   b. Victor's sperm, implanted in a surrogate mother.

   c. Victor's sperm, implanted in Ann after genetic restructuring.

   d. donor sperm, implanted in Victor's sterilized testes.

46. Briefly describe the following reproductive technologies:

   a. Artifical insemination

   b. In vitro fertilization (IVF)

   c. Gamete intrafallopian transfer (GIFT)

   d. Zygote intrafallopian transfer (ZIFT)

   e. Micromanipulation and blastomere analysis

47. As a nurse working in an office that focuses on infertility evaluation and treatment, it is your responsibility to coordinate care for couples, provide ongoing information and teaching, and evaluate the couple's psychosocial status. Dorothy Lewis, age 37, has had extensive testing and treatment in an effort to correct her infertility, but all approaches have failed. During a conversation with you, Dorothy expresses the feeling that she is a failure as a woman and a wife. She states, "We both think that children are an important part of marriage, but because of me, because my body can't do what it should, we are the losers. I am such a failure as a woman." Based on this information, formulate a possible nursing diagnosis that might apply.

48.   Identify some of the defining characteristics that led you to this diagnosis.

49.   For infertile couples, the most difficult aspect of their problem is likely to be the

    a.   financial burden.

    b.   emotional aspect.

    c.   painful and time-consuming testing.

    d.   decision to adopt or remain childless.

Genetic Disorders

50.   The pictorial analysis of an individual's chromosomes is called a _____.

51.   Tammy Daniel has cystic fibrosis. Because this is a condition of autosomal recessive inheritance, the nurse knows Tammy most likely inherited the disease from

    a.   her mother.

    b.   her father.

    c.   both parents, who are carriers of the abnormal gene.

    d.   neither parent, but as a result of a toxic environment in utero.

52.   Your client's husband, who was adopted as an infant, has just been diagnosed as having Huntington's chorea. Your client asks you what the possibility is that their two children will develop the disease. What is the correct answer? Diagram the pattern of inheritance demonstrating your rationale for your response.

53.   If one parent has cystic fibrosis and the other has normal genes, what is the probability that their children will have cystic fibrosis? Diagram your rationale for your response.

54.   Draw a family tree (pedigree) for your family as far back as your grandparents, if possible. Are there any conditions your family considers hereditary? Don't forget to include findings such as high blood pressure, obesity, and diabetes. If you are not familiar with drawing family trees (pedigrees), you may find it helpful to consult a physical assessment text.

55.   **Memory Check:** Define the following abbreviations.

a.   AF   d.   hCS

b.   BBT   e.   hMG

c.   hCG   f.   hPL

4 | Women's Health Care

This chapter corresponds to Chapter 5 in the 4th edition of *Maternal-Newborn Nursing Care: The Nurse, the Family, and the Community.*

The Role of the Nurse in Menstrual Counseling

Match the definitions listed on the right with the correct terms below.

1. __b__ Amenorrhea   a. Abnormally short menstrual cycle

2. __a__ Hypomenorrhea   b. Absence of menses

3. __c__ Menorrhagia   c. Excessive menstrual flow

4. __e__ Dysmenorrhea   d. Bleeding between periods

5. __f__ Hypermenorrhea   e. Painful menses

6. __d__ Metrorrhagia   f. Abnormally long menstrual cycle

7. Discuss premenstrual syndrome (PMS) with regard to etiology, signs and symptoms, and treatment. Include information on self-care measures women with PMS might employ.

Reflections

Some women view menstruation as a normal, even welcome, part of life; some women view it as a minor annoyance; some women are embarrassed by it; others consider it a "curse" and hate it. Take a few moments to explore your views on menstruation. Try to identify some of the factors that have influenced your attitudes about it.

_____

_____

_____

_____

_____

_____

_____

Contraceptive Methods

For each of the methods of contraception listed below, select the appropriate mechanism of action from the list on the right.

8.   _____b_____ Condom   a.   Prevents ovulation

9.   _____a_____ Norplant   b.   Prevents transport of sperm to the ovum

10.   _____b_____ Diaphragm

11.   _____a_____ Depo-Provera

12.   _____b_____ Oral contraceptive

13.   When using a diaphragm, the woman should use additional spermicide before intercourse if

      more than (a) _____4_____ hours have elapsed since the diaphragm was inserted. She should

      leave the diaphragm in place for at least (b) _____6_____ hours after intercourse.

14.   Marcella Taylor has two children by a previous marriage. She has just begun seeing a man and asks you if the IUD would be a good contraceptive method if they become sexually involved. How would you respond?

IUD is recommended who have given birth and sleep with 1 man. If he sleeps with other women he needs to wear a condom

15.   The male sterilization procedure is called (a) *vasectomy*; female sterilization is called (b) *tubal ligation*.

16.   An estrogen-related side effect of oral contraceptives is

    a.   acne.

    b.   decreased libido.

    c.   hirsutism.

    d.   hypertension.

Menopause

17.   Mrs Joan Sanchez, age 50, has been coming to this office for her gynecologic exams for the past 7 years. Last year, she mentioned some irregularity in her periods. During her annual physical exam and Pap smear, she tells you that her periods have been more irregular and her last period was about 3 months ago. In addition, she has been experiencing difficulty sleeping; a sense of heat rising over her chest, neck, and face; increased perspiration; and palpitations. You identify that Mrs Sanchez is entering menopause. In your counseling session, what information about self-care measures can you provide?

*Use fans
Cold liquids for hot flashes
Continue calcium supplement
Water soluble jelly during intercourse*

18. **Critical Thinking Challenge:** The following situation has been included to challenge your critical thinking. Read the situation and then answer the question "yes" or "no."

Yvonne Swenson, age 52, is being seen for her annual examination. Her history reveals that she is a slender woman of Swedish ancestry who completed menopause at age 46. She does not drink alcohol but does smoke three-fourths of a pack of cigarettes per day. She has two children.

Is Ms Swenson at increased risk of developing osteoporosis?

Yes _____   No _____

Explain your answer:

early onset of menopause.
fair complexion
smoker
slender built

19. In women who have a uterus and who are on hormone replacement therapy (HRT), the estrogen is opposed by giving (a) _____progestin_____ for all or part of the cycle to prevent the increased risk of developing (b) _____endometrial ca_____ .

20. Which of the following is a risk factor for osteoporosis?
    a. Black race
    b. Late onset of menopause
    c. Multiparity
    d. Thin and small-boned build

Violence Against Women

21. Identify at least four signs that may indicate a woman is experiencing female partner abuse.
    a. does not want to tell how an incident occurred. How she got bruised. delay reporting symptoms
    b. pattern of injury consistent with abuse. injuries in the head/back/neck
    c. ↑ anxiety when batterer is around
    d.

Match the definitions on the right with the type of rape they best describe.

22. _____c_____ Anger rape   a. Assailant is known to the victim; previously the
                                        relationship was nonviolent.

23. _____a_____ Confidence rape   b. Assailant wishes to feel dominant and typically uses only
                                        the force necessary to subdue his victim.

24. _____b_____ Power rape   c. Attack is used to express feelings of rage and is often
                                        brutal and degrading.

25. _____d_____ Sadistic rape   d. Planned assault characterized by torture, mutilation,
                                        and often murder.

26. Briefly describe the Sexual Assault Nurse Examiner (SANE) Program.

P119

The Female Breast

27. Annual mammograms are recommended for all women over age _____40_____.

Imagine you are responsible for teaching the correct procedure for monthly breast self-examination to healthy women.

28. Explain the purpose for visually inspecting the breasts with the arms in a variety of positions.

29. Explain the procedure for breast self-examination.

30. Which of the following findings during breast self-examination should a woman report to her health care provider?

    a. Difference in size between the breasts

    b. Silver-colored striae

    c. Symmetrical venous pattern

    d. Thickened skin with enlarged pores

31. Your client asks if there are any self-care measures she can use to attempt to decrease the discomfort she experiences cyclically because of fibrocystic breast disease. What advice would you give her?

Gynecologic Disorders

32. The three most common symptoms of endometriosis are

    a. _____pelvic____ _____pain____   b. _dyspareunia_   c. _abnormal uterine bleeding_

33. In the office where you work as a nurse, one of the women being treated for endometriosis is going to begin taking danazol. You assess her knowledge level and find that she has only a vague understanding of the medication. You formulate the nursing diagnosis: Knowledge deficit related to lack of information about the medication danazol. Based on this nursing diagnosis, what information would you give her about the drug?

34.   A primary side effect of danazol (Danocrine) is

     a.   dry, flaky skin.

     b.   hirsutism.

     c.   increased libido.

     d.   weight loss.

35.   Your client asks you about health practices she can follow to help her avoid developing toxic shock syndrome (TSS). What recommendations would you make?

Match the characteristic vaginal discharge listed on the right with the correct type of vaginitis.

36.   _c_   Bacterial vaginosis   a.   Greenish-white and frothy

37.   _a_   Trichomoniasis   b.   Thick, white, curdy

38.   _b_   Vulvovaginal candidiasis   c.   Gray, milky

39.   The presence of clue cells on a wet mount preparation is indicative of

     a.   bacterial vaginosis.

     b.   chlamydia.

     c.   trichomoniasis.

     d.   vulvovaginal candidiasis.

For each of the infections listed below, select the appropriate antibiotic treatment from the list on the right for a woman who is not pregnant.

40.   _b_   Chlamydia   a.   Benzathine penicillin G

41.   _d_   Gonorrhea   b.   Doxycycline

42.   _a_   Syphilis   c.   Clotrimazole

43.   _c_   Vulvovaginal candidiasis   b.   Ceftriaxone

44. **Critical Thinking in Practice:** The following action sequence is designed to help you think through clinical problems. Read the sequence below, then fill in the appropriate boxes in the flowchart that follows.

Imagine you work as a registered nurse in a women's health clinic. It is your responsibility to interview women initially and obtain data on the purpose of their visit. You also do health teaching. You do not do pelvic examinations. Nita Trujillo, a client at the clinic, tells you she is there today because she has had marked itching of her vulva and vagina. She states, "It itches so bad that I've scratched it raw and made it worse." She tells you she has never had a vaginal infection before and has not been sexually active for three months. She says that she has had no symptoms of a urinary tract infection although it does burn when the urine touches the excoriated skin.

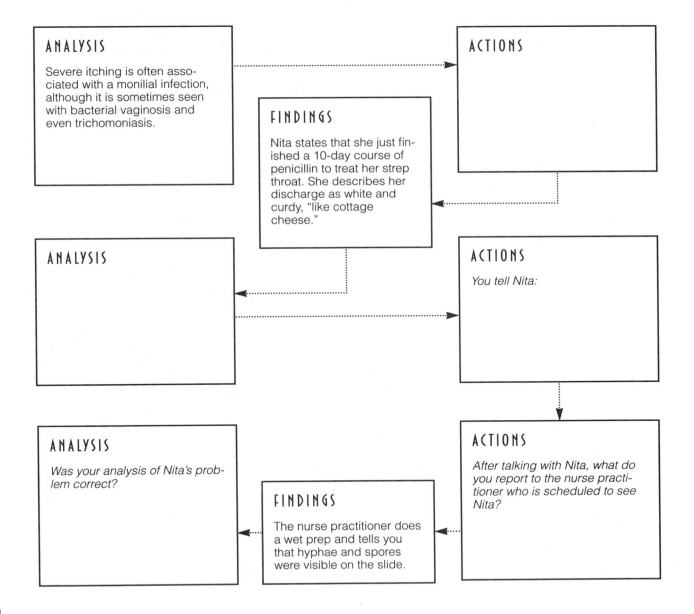

ANALYSIS

Severe itching is often associated with a monilial infection, although it is sometimes seen with bacterial vaginosis and even trichomoniasis.

ACTIONS

FINDINGS

Nita states that she just finished a 10-day course of penicillin to treat her strep throat. She describes her discharge as white and curdy, "like cottage cheese."

ANALYSIS

ACTIONS

You tell Nita:

ANALYSIS

Was your analysis of Nita's problem correct?

ACTIONS

After talking with Nita, what do you report to the nurse practitioner who is scheduled to see Nita?

FINDINGS

The nurse practitioner does a wet prep and tells you that hyphae and spores were visible on the slide.

45. Marcy D'Angelo, diagnosed with trichomoniasis, has been given prescriptions for metronidazole for her and her partner. In addition to general teaching about the medication, what specific warning should you give Marcy?

46. The greatest long-term problem caused by pelvic inflammatory disease (PID) is _____.

47. Compare cystitis and pyelonephritis:

	Cystitis	Pyelonephritis
Signs and symptoms		
Therapy		
Implications		
Client education		

48. **Memory Check:** Define the following abbreviations.

a. BBT

b. BSE

c. CDC

d. D&C

e. FBD

f. PID

g. STD

h. UTI

5 | Physical and Psychologic Changes of Pregnancy

This chapter corresponds to Chapter 7 in the 4th edition of *Maternal-Newborn Nursing Care: The Nurse, the Family, and the Community.*

Anatomy and Physiology of Pregnancy

1. The primary cause of uterine enlargement during pregnancy is the

    a. engorgement of pre-existing vascular structures.

    b. formation of an additional layer of uterine musculature.

    c. hypertrophy of pre-existing myometrial cells.

    d. increased number of myometrial cells.

2. How are the circulatory requirements of the uterus affected by pregnancy?

3. Many of the changes that occur in the pelvic organs during pregnancy are named. For each of the following changes, identify its correct name:

    a. The deep reddish-purple coloration of the mucosa of the cervix, vagina, and vulva is called ____Chadwick____ sign.

    b. The softening of the cervix that occurs is called ____Goodells____ sign.

    c. The softening of the isthmus of the uterus is called ____Hegar____ sign.

4. During pregnancy, the increased number and activity of the endocervical glands are responsible for

    a. a marked softening of the cervix.

    b. a thinner, more watery mucosal discharge.

    c. the development of Chadwick's sign.

    d. the formation of the mucous plug.

5. What function does the mucous plug serve?

    It prevent the asent of organisms from the vaginal tract into the uterus

6. The ovaries _____ stop _____ ovum production during pregnancy.

7. During the first 10–12 weeks of pregnancy, the corpus luteum

    a. gradually regresses and becomes obliterated.

    b. secretes estrogen to maintain the pregnancy.

    c. secretes human chorionic gonadotropin to maintain the pregnancy.

    d. secretes progesterone to maintain the pregnancy.

8. What is the significance of the increased acidity of the vaginal secretions during pregnancy?

    help prevent bacterial infections but favors the growth of yeast organism

9. Describe the breast changes that occur during pregnancy with regard to the following:

    a. Size ↑

    b. Pigmentation areolas darken

    c. Montgomery's tubercles become more pronounce and enlarged

10. Why is there an increased tendency toward nasal stuffiness and epistaxis during pregnancy?

    estrogen - induced edema and vascular congestion of the nasal mucosa

For the components of the cardiovascular system listed below, indicate whether there is normally an increase (**I**) or a decrease (**D**) during pregnancy.

11.   _____D_____ Blood pressure

12.   _____I_____ Erythrocyte volume

13.   _____I_____ Cardiac output

14.   _____D_____ Hematocrit

15.   _____I_____ Pulse

16.   The pseudoanemia of pregnancy is caused by

    a.   a greater increase in plasma volume than in hemoglobin levels.

    b.   decreased hemoglobin levels.

    c.   a decrease in both plasma volume and hemoglobin levels.

    (d.) increased plasma volume without a comparable increase in hemoglobin levels.

17.   During pregnancy, the enlarging uterus may cause pressure on the vena cava when the woman lies supine, interfering with returning blood flow. As a result the woman may feel dizzy and clammy, and her blood pressure may decrease. This condition is called the (a) _hypo sensitive_ syndrome or (b) _vena carval_ syndrome.

18.   Constipation during pregnancy is usually the result of

    (a.) prolonged stomach emptying time and decreased intestinal motility.

    b.   increased peristalsis and flatulence.

    c.   increased cardiac workload resulting in delayed peristalsis.

    d.   reflux of acidic gastric contents and hypochlorhydria.

19.   Identify the causes of each of the following discomforts of pregnancy:

    a.   Heartburn

    b.   Hemorrhoids

    c.   Urinary frequency

20. Which of the following changes in kidney functioning occurs during a normal pregnancy?

    a. Blood urea nitrogen values increase

    (b.) Glomerular filtration rate increases

    c. Renal plasma flow decreases

    d. Renal tubular reabsorption rate decreases

Many changes occur in the skin during pregnancy. Match the terms identifying these changes with their appropriate definition:

21. ____c___ Chloasma   a. Line of darker pigmentation extending from the pubis to the umbilicus in some women

22. ____d___ Striae gravidarum   b. Small, bright red, vascular elevations of the skin often found on the chest, arms, legs, and neck

23. ____b___ Spider nevi   c. The "mask of pregnancy," an irregular pigmentation commonly found on the cheeks, forehead, and nose

24. ____a___ Linea nigra   d. Wavy, irregular, reddish streaks commonly found on the abdomen, breasts, or thighs; often referred to as "stretch marks"

25. A pregnant woman tells you that her friends tease her about her "stomach-first, waddling walk." She asks why she walks this way. How would you respond?

26. Briefly describe the functions of the following hormones in pregnancy:

    a. Human chorionic gonadotropin (hCG)

    b. Estrogen

   c.   Progesterone

   d.   Human placental lactogen (hPL)

   e.   Relaxin

27.   Briefly discuss the proposed functions of prostaglandins during pregnancy.

28.   Describe the effects of pregnancy on the following components of the endocrine system:

   a.   Thyroid

   b.   Pancreas

   c.   Pituitary

   d.   Adrenals

29.   What is the recommended weight gain for a woman of normal weight before pregnancy?

30.   What is the average pattern of weight gain during each trimester of pregnancy?

    a.   First trimester:

    b.   Second trimester:

    c.   Third trimester:

For each of the following signs of pregnancy, indicate with an **S, O,** or **D** whether the sign is subjective (presumptive), objective (probable), or diagnostic (positive).

31.   _____   Amenorrhea

32.   _____   Goodell's sign

33.   _____   Fetal heart sounds

34.   _____   Urinary frequency

35.   _____   Positive pregnancy test

36.   _____   Nausea and vomiting

37.   _____   Enlargement of the abdomen

38.   _____   Quickening

39.   _____   Palpable fetal movements

40.   _____   Braxton Hicks contractions

41.   How would you explain the differences among subjective (presumptive), objective (probable), and diagnostic (positive) signs of pregnancy to an expectant mother?

Pregnancy Tests

42.   Briefly describe each of the following pregnancy tests:

    a.   Hemagglutination-inhibition test (Pregnosticon R)

    b.   Latex agglutination tests (Gravindex and Pregnosticon slide test)

    c.   Beta subunit radioimmunoassay (RIA)

    d.   Enzyme-linked immunosorbent assay (ELISA)

    e.   Immunoradiometric assay (IRMA)

    f.   Radioreceptor assay (RRA) (Biocept G)

43.   Why is a positive pregnancy test *not* a positive sign of pregnancy?

44.   Over-the-counter pregnancy tests determine the presence of hCG in the woman's

    a.   blood.

    b.   saliva.

    c.   urine.

    d.   vaginal secretions.

Psychologic Response of the Expectant Family to Pregnancy

45.   Briefly summarize behaviors that are commonly seen in each trimester as a woman adjusts
to pregnancy.

Trimester	Behaviors
First trimester	
Second trimester	
Third trimester	

46.   Discuss the possible effects of pregnancy on a woman's body image.

47.   Rubin (1984) suggests that a pregnant woman faces four main psychologic tasks as she works
to maintain her intactness and that of her family while also preparing a place for her new child.
Identify and briefly summarize these tasks.

    a.

b.

c.

d.

Reflections

Think of some pregnant women you have known or cared for who were at different stages of pregnancy. How did their responses to pregnancy vary? What feelings did they describe? How did their partners react? Their parents? Other children in the family?

_____

_____

_____

_____

_____

_____

_____

_____

48. As her pregnancy progresses, Alana Lewis begins to see less of the women in her Young Businesswomen's Club and spends more time with two neighbors who have young children. Which of Rubin's psychologic tasks of pregnancy is she attempting to complete?

    a. Ensuring safe passage through pregnancy, labor, and birth

    b. Seeking of acceptance of this child by others

    c. Seeking of commitment and acceptance of self as mother to the infant

    d. Learning to give of self on behalf of child

49. Your close friend has just received confirmation that she is 10 weeks pregnant. She tells you that she feels some ambivalence about being pregnant and having a child, even though the pregnancy was planned. How might you respond?

50. Like the pregnant woman, the reactions of the expectant father to pregnancy tend to vary by trimester. For each trimester, describe the commonly occurring responses of the father.

    First trimester:

    Second trimester:

    Third trimester:

51. Briefly explain the concept of couvade.

52. Monica Clark is 6 months pregnant and asks for advice about how to prepare her 3-year-old son Jared for the birth of a sibling. What suggestions might you give her?

53. Imagine you are the head nurse in a prenatal clinic that provides care for women from a variety of ethnic backgrounds. You are responsible for orienting new nurses. Summarize three or four key points for the nurses to remember when caring for women from different cultures.

54. **Memory Check:** Define the following abbreviations.

a. hCG

b. hPL

6 Nursing Assessment and Care of the Expectant Family

This chapter corresponds to Chapters 6, 8, 9, 10, and 11 in the 4th edition of *Maternal-Newborn Nursing Care: The Nurse, the Family, and the Community.*

Preparation for Childbirth

1. Define *birth plan*.

2. During pregnancy, the expectant family begins to plan for their childbirth experience. Identify at least six issues a family should consider in their decision making.

   a.

   b.

   c.

   d.

   e.

   f.

3. Compare the psychoprophylactic (Lamaze) method of childbirth preparation to a method commonly used in your area with regard to philosophy and basic approaches.

Prenatal Assessment

Match the terms on the left, which are used when developing a woman's obstetric history, with the definitions on the right:

4. __d__   Gravida

    a. A woman who has had two or more births at more than 20 weeks' gestation

5. __a__   Multipara

    b. A woman who has never been pregnant

6. __b__   Nulligravida

    c. A woman who is pregnant for the first time

7. __f__   Para

    d. Any pregnancy, regardless of its duration, including the present pregnancy

8. __c__   Primigravida

    e. A woman who has not given birth at more than 20 weeks' gestation

    f. Birth after 20 weeks' gestation, regardless of whether the infant is born alive or dead

9. Alexis Page is pregnant for the fourth time. She lost her first pregnancy at 12 weeks' gestation. She has two children at home. How would you record her obstetric history?

Gravida _____   Para _____   Ab _____   Living children _____

10. a. Kerry Lawrence is pregnant for the third time. She gave birth to a stillborn infant at 36 weeks' gestation and has a 3-year-old at home who was born at term. How would you record her obstetric history?

Gravida _____   Para _____   Ab _____   Living children _____

b. A more detailed approach can also be used. In this approach, the meaning of *gravida* remains unchanged while *para* changes slightly to focus on the number of infants born. Use the acronym TPAL to remember *T*erm, *P*reterm, *A*bortions, *L*iving children. Using this method, how would you record Kerry's obstetric history?

Gravida _____   Para ____ ____ ____ ____

11. The following questionnaire is similar to many that are used when a woman initially seeks antepartal care. With a friend or family member acting as the client and you as the prenatal nurse, obtain the necessary information. (Note: This questionnaire focuses primarily on factors related to pregnancy and is not a complete history of all body systems.)

Name: _____   Age: _____   Race: _____

Address: _____   Phone: _____

Educational level: _____   Occupation: _____

Marital status: _____   Religious preference (optional) _____

→

Questionnaire, continued

Have any members of your family had the following? If so, who?

_____ Diabetes _____

_____ Cardiovascular disease _____

_____ High blood pressure _____

_____ Breast cancer _____

_____ Other types of cancer _____

_____ Multiple pregnancies _____

_____ Preeclampsia-eclampsia (pregnancy-induced hypertension) _____

_____ Congenital anomalies _____

How old were you when your menstrual periods started? _____

How often do they occur? _____

How long do they last? _____

Do you have any discomfort with your periods? _____ If so, how severe is it? _____

What is the date of the first day of your last normal menstrual period? _____

Have you had any bleeding or spotting since your last normal menstrual period? _____

Have you had any of the following diseases?

_____ Chickenpox	_____ Asthma
_____ Mumps	_____ High blood pressure
_____ Three-day measles (rubella)	_____ Heart disease
_____ Two-week measles (rubeola)	_____ Respiratory disease
_____ Kidney disease	_____ Diabetes
_____ Frequent bladder infections	_____ Allergies
_____ Thyroid problems	_____ Sexually transmitted infection
_____ Anemia	_____ Other

(If the woman answers *yes* to any of the above, include pertinent information in this space.)

Have you been on birth control pills? _____ If yes, when did you stop taking them? _____

Were you using any other method of contraception? _____ If so, what method? _____

How many previous pregnancies have you had? _____

Have you had any miscarriages or abortions? _____ If yes, how many? _____

How many living children do you have? _____

Have you had any stillbirths? _____ If yes, how many? _____

Gravida _____ Para _____ Ab _____

Previous children:

	Date of birth	Sex	Birth weight	Preterm or full term
1.				
2.				
3.				
4.				
5.				

Did any previous children have problems immediately after birth? _____ If yes, what occurred?

Have you had any problems with previous pregnancies? _____ If yes, what occurred?

Have you had any problems with previous labors and/or births? _____ If yes, what occurred?

Have you had any problems with previous postpartal periods? _____ If yes, what occurred?

Are you presently taking any prescription or nonprescription drugs? _____ If yes, please list them:

Do you smoke? _____ Number of cigarettes per day: _____

How much of the following do you drink each day? Coffee _____ Tea _____

Colas _____ Alcoholic beverages _____

What is your present weight? _____ What is your usual prepregnant weight? _____

Questionnaire, continued

Nursing assessment of available psychosocial data (*to be completed by nurse using information obtained from the woman or other sources*):[1]

Brief description of available support persons (include information about the father of the child such as age, occupation, involvement in the pregnancy):

Client feelings about the pregnancy and her plans for dealing with it:

Does the client have any cultural or religious practices that might influence her care or that of her child?

For the prenatal laboratory test results listed below, indicate with an **N** if the result is normal or an **A** if the result is abnormal and requires further evaluation.

12. _____ Hemoglobin 13.6 g/dL

13. _____ Hematocrit 35%

14. _____ Rubella titer 1:6

15. _____ WBC 6,200/ L

16. _____ Sickle cell screen negative

[1]This should be a brief summary of your impression of the woman, her ability to cope with her pregnancy, plans she has made, and available support systems.

17.   During the prenatal assessment, the woman is screened for risk factors. What are risk factors?

18.   Give three examples of factors that increase a woman's risk.

    a.

    b.

    c.

The procedure for a complete physical examination may be reviewed in textbooks on physical assessment. This workbook focuses on those aspects of the physical examination that are directly related to assessment of the pregnancy.

19.   Allison Scott, gravida 1 para 0 ab 0, is scheduled for her first obstetric examination. Identify three areas of focus in this examination.

    a.

    b.

    c.

20.   During her examination, the nurse practitioner (or physician) measures Allison's fundal height. How is this measured?

21.   a.   What information does fundal height provide about the pregnancy?

    b.   Where would you expect to find the fundus at 12 weeks' gestation? _____

    c.   At 20 weeks' gestation?_____

22.   Allison asks you when the baby's heartbeat will be heard. When is the fetal heartbeat usually detected?

    a.   With a fetoscope: _____

    b.   With a Doppler: _____

23.   To complete a pelvic examination, Allison is placed in the _____ position.

24.   Identify the three basic parts of every initial pelvic examination.

    a.

    b.

    c.

25.   If you noted on a prenatal record that a woman had a diagonal conjugate of 9.0 cm, what possible problems might you predict for her labor?

26.   What is the purpose of Nägele's rule?

27.   How is Nägele's rule calculated?

28.   Allison began her last normal menstrual period on March 22 of this year. Using Nägele's rule, calculate her expected date of birth (EDB).

29.   What is the recommended frequency of prenatal visits for a normal prenatal client?

30.   Identify the factors that you would consider part of your initial psychologic assessment of an antepartal family.

For each of the warning signs listed below, select a possible cause from the choices on the right. Use each answer only once.

31.   _____ Dysuria   a.   Preeclampsia

32.   _____ Persistent vomiting   b.   Placenta previa

33.   _____ Abdominal pain   c.   Urinary tract infection

34.   _____ Epigastric pain   b.   Hyperemesis gravidarum

35.   _____ Vaginal bleeding   c.   Abruptio placentae

36.   What would you instruct a woman to do if she experiences any of the danger signs in pregnancy?

Common Discomforts of Pregnancy

37.   From the list that follows, circle the discomforts that commonly occur during the first trimester of pregnancy:

varicose veins, urinary frequency, nausea and vomiting,

backache, dyspnea, flatulence, fatigue, leg cramps,

breast tenderness, faintness, increased vaginal discharge

38.   For each of the discomforts listed below, identify at least one self-care measure a pregnant woman might use to obtain relief.

   a.   Breast tenderness

   b.   Leg cramps

   c.   Nausea

   d.   Constipation

   e.   Backache

   f.   Urinary frequency

39.   Your friend is in her early months of pregnancy and complains about morning sickness. Which of the following recommendations might you make to her?

   a.   Nothing will alleviate it, and you must do your best to accept it.

   b.   Eat a dry carbohydrate, such as crackers, before arising.

   c.   Take large quantities of fluids with meals.

   d.   Eat three meals per day and avoid eating between meals.

40.   **Critical Thinking in Practice:** The following action sequence is designed to help you think through basic clinical problems. Read the sequence below, then fill in the appropriate boxes in the flowchart on page 59.

   Jan Lynd, G1 P0, is 12 weeks pregnant when she comes for her second prenatal visit. She tells you that her main problem is noticeable fatigue. She states, "Sometimes I'm so tired by the end of the day that I can hardly make it home to cook supper. I can't tell you how many meals Larry has cooked lately because I don't have the energy to do it. Is something wrong with me?"

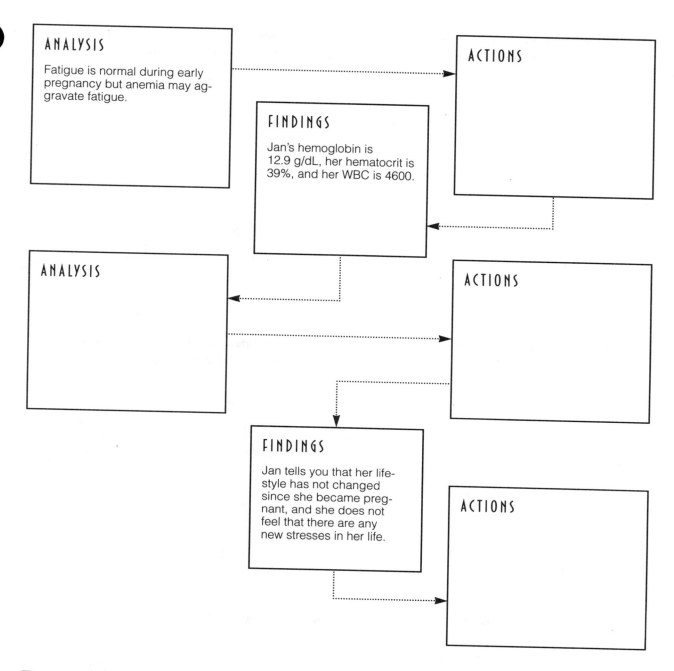

Prenatal Teaching

41.   Mary Jo Bryant is interested in breastfeeding her baby and asks if there is anything she should do during pregnancy to prepare her breasts. What advice would you give her?

42. Mary Jo asks about the types of physical activity she can engage in during pregnancy. What guidelines would you suggest she follow when engaging in sports and physical activities?

43. Several approaches to tracking fetal activity exist and are often referred to as a fetal movement record or fetal activity diary. Describe the procedure for tracking fetal activity that is used in your clinical facility.

44. Linh Trang, 7 months pregnant, asks about traveling 300 miles by car to visit her parents. Her pregnancy, to date, is normal. What advice would you give her?

45. What advice would you give a pregnant woman who states that she is a "bath person" and prefers tub baths to showers?

46. The pregnant woman should have a dental examination (a) _____ in her

    pregnancy. Dental x-rays should be (b) _____ .

47. What advice would you give a woman 11 weeks pregnant who asks about having an occasional glass of wine during her pregnancy?

48. Kathy Wilson is 7 months pregnant with her first child. She tells you that she and her partner, Chuck, still find sexual intercourse very satisfying, although recently they have found it more comfortable to make love if Kathy assumes the superior position. Kathy says that she and Chuck recently talked about making love during the last weeks of pregnancy. They wondered if it was "okay" or if it posed a threat for Kathy or the baby. After assessing Kathy's concerns, formulate an appropriate nursing diagnosis.

Age-Related Considerations

49. Identify at least six reasons why an adolescent might become pregnant.

    a.

    b.

    c.

    d.

    e.

    f.

Reflections

Think about any pregnant adolescents you have cared for as a nursing student or have known. Compare their reactions to being pregnant to those of more mature pregnant women. How are they similar? Different?

_____

_____

_____

_____

_____

_____

_____

_____

50.   Imagine you are responsible for developing a prenatal clinic for adolescent girls. What factors about the adolescent and her development would you consider in planning your approach? Identify some specific techniques or services you would like to have available for the adolescent.

51. For the pregnant adolescent, the most common medical complication is

   a. gestational diabetes mellitus.

   b. herpes simplex.

   c. pregnancy-induced hypertension.

   d. pyelonephritis.

52. A child born to a woman over age 35 has an increased risk of

   a. Down syndrome.

   b. cleft palate.

   c. cystic fibrosis.

   d. meningomyelocele.

Maternal Nutrition

53. Diana Cooper, a 22-year-old primipara, 2 months pregnant, is discussing nutrition with you. She is of normal weight and is very concerned about avoiding excessive weight gain. What pattern of weight gain would you recommend for her?

54. To achieve this weight gain, she should increase her daily intake by _____ kcal.

55. Which of the following menus would provide the highest amounts of protein, iron, and vitamin C?

   a. 4 oz beef, ½ c lima beans, a glass of skim milk, and ¾ c strawberries

   b. 3 oz chicken, ½ c corn, a lettuce salad, and a small banana

   c. 1 c macaroni, ¾ c peas, a glass of whole milk, and a medium pear

   d. A scrambled egg, hashbrown potatoes, half a glass of buttermilk, and a large nectarine

For each of the vitamins or minerals listed below, select the answer that best describes their function from the column on the right.

56. _____ Vitamin A   a. Prevents night blindness

57. _____ Vitamin E   b. Necessary for normal blood clotting

58. _____ Vitamin K   c. Essential to formation of connective tissue

59. _____ Vitamin C   d. Synthesis of DNA and RNA

60. _____ Folic acid   e. Amino acid metabolism

61. _____ Pyridoxine (B$_6$) f. Cellular metabolism

62. _____ Calcium   g. Deficiency associated with neural tube defects

63. _____ Zinc   h. Mineralization of fetal bones and teeth

64. _____ Magnesium   i. Antioxidation

65. Tina Nelson is a true vegetarian and will not eat any food from animal sources, including milk and eggs. What foods might she use to meet her protein and calcium requirements during pregnancy?

66. The following is a 24-hour food diary for a 26-year-old pregnant woman of normal weight. Analyze its adequacy with regard to the basic food groups.

Breakfast:

¾ oz dry cereal

½ cup lowfat milk

4 oz orange juice

Lunch:

sandwich made with 2 slices whole wheat bread, 2 oz chicken breast, lettuce, mayonnaise

8 oz milk

1 small chocolate bar

Dinner:

6 oz flounder

tossed salad with dressing

½ cup rice

1 piece of cake

Snack:

1½ cup vanilla ice cream

Analysis:

Dairy products:

Meat group:

Grains:

Fruits and vegetables:

67.   **Memory Check:** Define the following abbreviations.

a.   EDB

b.   EDC

c.   EDD

d.   FAD

e.   FMR

f.   G

g.   P

h.   RDA

7 | Pregnancy at Risk: Pregestational Problems

This chapter corresponds to Chapter 12 in the 4th edition of *Maternal-Newborn Nursing Care: The Nurse, the Family, and the Community.*

Heart Disease and Pregnancy

1. The New York Heart Association classification of functional capacity is used to assess the severity of cardiac disease. For each of the classes, state the expected physical activity level.

   a. Class I

   b. Class II

   c. Class III

   d. Class IV

2. Sandy Carson is a 24-year-old woman who is classified as a class III cardiac client. List five signs and symptoms that would lead you to suspect cardiac decompensation in Sandy.

   a.

   b.

   c.

d.

e.

3. Juanita Alvarez has a history of cardiac problems following an episode of rheumatic fever. She experiences dyspnea and palpitations when she bicycles around her neighborhood. Which classification of functional capacity best applies?

    a. Class I

    b. Class II

    c. Class III

    d. Class IV

4. Which of the following statements about the nutritional needs of pregnant women with a cardiac condition is most accurate?

    a. They require major increases in iron and calories but decreased sodium.

    b. They require increased protein and iron but minimized sodium intake.

    c. They require optimal amounts of all essential vitamins but restricted caloric and iron intake.

    d. They require increased iron, protein, sodium, carbohydrates, and fats.

5. Amy Chang, 10 weeks pregnant, is seen for her first prenatal visit. She had rheumatic fever as a child and is currently classified as a class II cardiac client. In addition to iron and vitamin supplements, Amy is started on penicillin. She asks you why this was done. What would you tell her?

6. In the absence of complications, what is the method of choice by which Amy would give birth?

Diabetes Mellitus and Pregnancy

7. The four cardinal signs and symptoms of diabetes are

    a. _____   c. _____

    b. _____   d. _____

8. Mary Lewis is pregnant for the second time. Her first child weighed 9 lb 11 oz. Her doctors perform a glucose tolerance test and discover elevated blood glucose levels. Because Mary shows no signs of diabetes when she is not pregnant, she is best classified as having

    a. type I diabetes mellitus.

    b. type II diabetes mellitus.

    c. gestational diabetes mellitus.

    d. secondary diabetes mellitus.

9. Following birth, the infant of a woman with type I diabetes mellitus is at greatest risk for the development of

    a. anemia.

    b. hypercalcemia.

    c. hyperglycemia.

    d. hypoglycemia.

10. Identify three ways in which pregnancy can affect diabetes.

    a.

    b.

    c.

11. Identify four maternal and/or fetal complications that may occur during pregnancy as a result of diabetes mellitus.

    a. _____   c. _____

    b. _____   d. _____

12. **Critical Thinking Challenge:** The following situation has been included to challenge your critical thinking. Read the situation and then answer "yes" or "no" to question on page 69.

    Belle Arthur, a 29-year-old G2 P1, was diagnosed as having diabetes mellitus a year ago. Her diabetes was controlled with low doses of insulin. When her pregnancy was diagnosed at 7 weeks' gestation, her glycosylated hemoglobin was 6.4% and her fasting blood glucose (FBG) was 98 mg/dL. Belle missed her last two prenatal visits but states that she carefully followed her diet and insulin dosage schedule. Today's FBG is 102 mg/dL and her glycosylated hemoglobin is 7.0%.

Did Ms Arthur maintain effective control?

Yes _____   No _____

Explain your answer:

13. You ask Ms Arthur if she can think of anything that would make it easier for her to keep her appointments. She states, "There is a satellite clinic really close to my house, but they won't see me because they say I'm high risk." You know that Belle's physician works at that clinic one day a week. You explain the situation and ask if she would be willing to see Belle there. The physician agrees, and Belle is delighted with the change. Evaluate the effectiveness of your intervention.

14. Isadora Fleming has newly diagnosed gestational diabetes and is started on insulin in two doses, one in the morning and one before dinner. She asks why two shots are necessary. How would you respond?

15. What advice would you give Isadora about continuing her regular exercise program?

16. Is breastfeeding safe for women with diabetes?

    a. yes

    b. no

17. A friend of yours is diagnosed as having gestational diabetes. She tells you that her grandmother takes tolbutamide (Orinase) for diabetes. Your friend asks why she can't simply take tolbutamide too. What would you tell her?

18.　Your friend also asks why infants of diabetic mothers are often large at birth. How would you explain this phenomenon?

19.　List three tests that might be performed to assess fetal status in a pregnant woman with diabetes.

　　a.

　　b.

　　c.

HIV Infection and Pregnancy

20.　The risk of HIV infection in infants born to women who are HIV-positive is about (a) _____ percent. The prenatal use of the medication (b) _____ by HIV-positive women helps reduce the risk of fetal transmission significantly.

21.　Identify four signs of developing complications in a pregnant HIV-positive woman.

　　a. _____　　c. _____

　　b. _____　　d. _____

22.　In caring for any pregnant woman, when should gloves be worn?

23.　According to CDC guidelines, which of the following statements about glove use is most accurate when caring for a newly born infant?

　　a.　Gloves are necessary only for invasive procedures.

　　b　Gloves are not required.

　　c.　Gloves should be worn at all times.

　　d.　Gloves should be worn until the admission bath is done.

ⓡeflections

HIV/AIDS is a devastating diagnosis for childbearing women and their loved ones. How do you feel about caring for families with HIV/AIDS? Do you have any preconceived views? Take a few moments to reflect on your own beliefs and attitudes. Do they influence the care you give?

_____

_____

_____

_____

_____

_____

_____

24. The most common method of HIV transmission for women is

    a. heterosexual activity.

    b. homosexual activity.

    c. intravenous drug use.

    d. travel to countries where HIV is endemic.

Substance Abuse and Pregnancy

For each of the substances listed below, identify at least one possible effect on the fetus of maternal use during pregnancy:

25. Alcohol

26. Cocaine/crack

27. Heroin

28.   **Memory Check:** Define the following abbreviations.

   a.   AIDS

   b.   DM

   c.   FAS

   d.   GDM

   e.   HIV

   f.   IDDM

8 | Pregnancy at Risk: Gestational Onset

This chapter corresponds to Chapter 13 in the 4th edition of *Maternal-Newborn Nursing Care: The Nurse, the Family, and the Community.*

Hyperemesis Gravidarum

1. Excessive vomiting during pregnancy is termed *hyperemesis gravidarum.* Identify the goals of therapy in treating a pregnant woman hospitalized with hyperemesis gravidarum.

Bleeding Disorders

Match the terms below with the correct definitions:

2. _____ Threatened abortion

    a. Loss of three or more successive pregnancies

3. _____ Imminent abortion

    b. Abortion characterized by vaginal bleeding and cramping but a closed cervical os

4. _____ Complete abortion

    c. Abortion in which the fetus dies in utero but is not expelled

5. _____ Incomplete abortion

    d. Abortion in which all the products of conception are expelled

6. _____ Missed abortion

    e. Abortion characterized by bleeding, cramping, and dilatation of the cervical os

7. _____ Habitual abortion

    f. Abortion in which a portion of the products of conception is retained

8. Alys Roberts, a 22-year-old gravida 1 para 0, 11 weeks pregnant, was admitted to the hospital with moderate vaginal bleeding and some abdominal cramping. Vaginal examination reveals that the cervix is dilated 2 cm. She is diagnosed as having an imminent abortion. Identify four nursing interventions that are indicated in caring for Alys.

    a.

    b.

    c.

    d.

9. Alys is placed on bed rest with intravenous fluids and that evening passes some of the products of conception. The following morning she has a dilation and curettage (D&C). Why is this done?

10. Alys' husband asks you why abortions occur. Identify four causes of spontaneous abortion.

    a.

    b.

    c.

    d.

11. The most common cause of second-trimester abortion is incompetent cervix. Identify two factors that may contribute to incompetent cervix.

    a.

    b.

12. A surgical procedure used to treat incompetent cervix so that a woman may successfully carry a pregnancy to term is _____.

13.   Define *ectopic pregnancy*.

14.   The most common implantation site in an ectopic pregnancy is the _____ .

15.   Ectopic pregnancy is often difficult to diagnose because its symptoms are similar to those of abdominal conditions. Identify at least five signs or symptoms of ectopic pregnancy and briefly explain why each occurs.

Sign or Symptom	Physiologic Rationale for Occurrence
a.	
b.	
c.	
d.	
e.	

16.   Which of the following signs would *not* be indicative of a ruptured tubal pregnancy?

a.   Marked lower abdominal pain

b.   Vaginal bleeding

c.   Urinary frequency

d.   Increased pulse and decreased blood pressure

17.   Which of the following findings would best support a diagnosis of gestational trophoblastic disease?

    a.   Elevated hCG levels, enlarged abdomen, quickening

    b.   Vaginal bleeding, absence of fetal heart tones, decreased hCG levels

    c.   Visible fetal skeleton with sonography, absence of quickening, enlarged abdomen

    d.   Brownish vaginal discharge, hyperemesis gravidarum, absence of fetal heart tones

18.   Lisa Chan is diagnosed as having gestational trophoblastic disease. Following successful removal of the molar pregnancy, Ms Chan is advised to avoid pregnancy for a year and to return for periodic measurement of human chorionic gonadotropin (hCG) levels. What is the rationale for this advice?

Preterm Labor

Sarah Smythe is 36 years old and is a gravida 4. She has two children at home; one was born at 35 weeks' gestation. Sarah had one spontaneous abortion. She smokes 15 cigarettes a day and has an occasional glass of wine. Sarah has a history of pyelonephritis. She has been working for the past 2 years in a factory. She provides the sole financial support for the family. Her job requires that she stand in one place along a conveyor belt and inspect parts as they pass by. Sarah had a brief episode of vaginal bleeding at 14 weeks' gestation, which lasted 2 days. Since then, the pregnancy has gone well; however, she has noted more contractions lately.

19.   In the narrative above, circle all of Mrs Smythe's risk factors for preterm labor.

20.   Mrs Smythe asks you what she should look for this time. Identify important information to include in your answer.

21. Mrs Smythe receives your information in a serious, thoughtful manner. At the end of your conversation, she says, "But how do I know if it's a real contraction?" What assessment techniques will you teach her?

There are many signs and symptoms associated with preterm labor. When any of the signs and symptoms of preterm labor are present, it is important for the woman to call her health care provider and be evaluated in a health care birth setting. Place an "X" beside all factors in the following list that would need further evaluation:

22. _____ nausea   26. _____ headache (mild) relieved by resting and cool cloth to forehead

23. _____ diarrhea   27. _____ backache

24. _____ thirst   28. _____ unusual tiredness

25. _____ cramps in legs   29. _____ increased appetite

30. Mrs Smythe is admitted in preterm labor at 30 weeks' gestation and is started on intravenous magnesium sulfate ($MgSO_4$). How does this medication work to control preterm labor?

31. The normal loading dose of $MgSO_4$ in treating preterm labor is (a) _____ g per infusion pump. The maintenance dose is (b) _____ g/hr per infusion pump.

32. The antagonist of $MgSO_4$ is _____ .

33.   When MgSO₄ is administered, careful nursing assessments are indicated. Identify at least five nursing assessments, the findings that would require further nursing action, and the rationale for each:

ASSESSMENT AND FINDINGS REQUIRING FURTHER ACTION	RATIONALE

34. **Critical Thinking Challenge:** The following situation has been included to challenge your critical thinking. Read the situation and then answer the question "yes" or "no."

   a. Mrs Quick is admitted to the birthing unit, and you will be responsible for her care. She is a G4, P3, ab 0, living children 3, term birth 1, preterm births 2. She is at 34 weeks' gestation and is having contractions every 3 minutes of 40 seconds duration. She states that her membranes have been ruptured since yesterday at noon (23 hours ago). In your initial assessments, you find FHR 140, T 99.2, P 92, R 18, cervical dilatation 5 cm, and Nitrazine positive.

   <u>**Is Mrs Quick a candidate for treatment to stop labor?**</u>

   Yes _____   No _____

   Explain your answer:

35. Mrs Aguilar is admitted in preterm labor at 32 weeks' gestation. In the first few minutes of care, many nursing actions are needed. Rank the nursing actions in order of priority. Place NA (not applicable) by those actions that could be deleted at this time.

   a. _____   Apply electronic monitor to determine contraction frequency and duration and FHR

   b. _____   Assess maternal B/P, TPR

   c. _____   Complete all sections of the admission form

   d. _____   Do a sterile vaginal examination to determine dilatation, effacement, fetal station, presentation, and position

   e. _____   Use Nitrazine to test for ruptured membranes

   f. _____   Weigh Mrs Aguilar

   g. _____   Listen to breath sounds

Pregnancy-Induced Hypertension (PIH)

36.   **Critical Thinking in Practice:** The following action sequence is designed to help you think through clinical problems.

You work as a professional nurse in a private obstetrician's office. Rita George, G1 P0, 37 weeks pregnant, is in for her weekly prenatal appointment. When you weigh her you note that she has gained 2¾ lb since last week. Her pregnancy to date has been completely normal. You know that the average weight gain in the last trimester is about 1 lb/week. A large weight gain often indicates that fluid is being retained. You know that this is an early sign of preeclampsia.

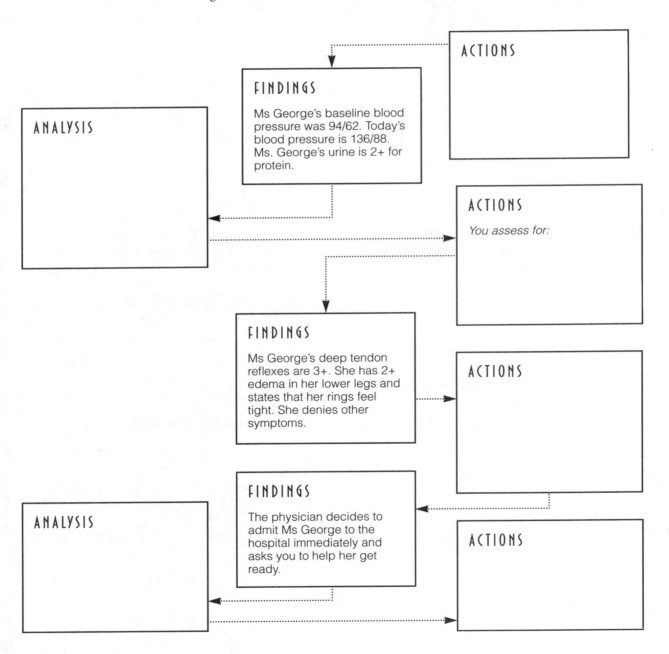

ACTIONS

FINDINGS

Ms George's baseline blood pressure was 94/62. Today's blood pressure is 136/88. Ms. George's urine is 2+ for protein.

ANALYSIS

ACTIONS

You assess for:

FINDINGS

Ms George's deep tendon reflexes are 3+. She has 2+ edema in her lower legs and states that her rings feel tight. She denies other symptoms.

ACTIONS

FINDINGS

The physician decides to admit Ms George to the hospital immediately and asks you to help her get ready.

ANALYSIS

ACTIONS

37.   On the following chart, compare the signs and symptoms of mild preeclampsia and severe preeclampsia (pregnancy-induced hypertension):

Sign	Mild Preeclampsia	Severe Preeclampsia
Blood pressure		
Weight gain		
Edema		
Proteinuria		
Hyperreflexia		
Headache		
Epigastric pain		
Visual disturbances		

38.   What additional symptom characterizes a woman as having eclampsia rather than severe preeclampsia? _____.

39.   Women with a diagnosis of severe preeclampsia have an increased risk of

a.   complete abortion.

b.   placenta previa.

c.   abruptio placentae.

d.   none of the above.

40.   Rita George is hospitalized with severe preeclampsia. Identify five interventions commonly
       used in caring for a woman with preeclampsia and the rationale for each.

Intervention	Rationale
a.	
b.	
c.	
d.	
e.	

41.   You are administering intravenous magnesium sulfate to a woman with severe preeclampsia.
       You assess her and find respirations 12, DTRs (deep tendon reflexes) absent, urine output for
       the past 4 hours of 90 mL. What would you do?

       a.   Administer calcium gluconate immediately.

       b.   Administer only half the dose of magnesium sulfate.

       c.   Continue the magnesium sulfate as ordered.

       d.   Stop the magnesium sulfate and notify the doctor.

42.   Your client, diagnosed with severe preeclampsia, is started on magnesium sulfate intravenously.

       In treating PIH, the normal loading dose of $MgSO_4$ is (a) _____ g given in a 20% solution

       via infusion pump over (b) _____ minutes. The maintenance dose is (c) _____ g/hour

       via infusion pump.

43.   Three signs of magnesium toxicity are (a) _____, (b) _____,

       and (c) _____.

44.   HELLP syndrome is a major complication of PIH. What do the letters HELLP stand for?

       H_____ E_____ L_____ L_____ P_____.

45.   Deborah Grand is admitted to the birthing center in active labor with her first pregnancy. Her blood pressure is now 140/86 (blood pressure at first prenatal visit was 110/66); she has 2+ pitting edema in her feet, ankles, and lower legs, and says that she has gained 4 pounds over the last 2 days. You check her patellar deep tendon reflexes (DTR). What does 3+ DTR mean?

46.   As you check DTR, you also assess clonus. How will you do this? What does 2 beats of clonus mean?

Rh Incompatibility

47.   **Critical Thinking Challenge:** The following situation has been developed to challenge your critical thinking. Read the situation and then answer the question "yes" or "no."

Your client, Carolyn Lorenzo, G2 P2, is Rh−; her partner is Rh+. Her first child was Rh−. She has just given birth to an Rh+ infant. Her indirect Coombs' test is positive. Her infant's direct Coombs' test is also positive.

Is Carolyn a candidate for Rh immune globulin (RhoGAM)?

Yes _____   No _____

Explain your answer:

48.   What does Rh immune globulin do?

49.   Briefly summarize the major risks for a woman and her fetus if the woman suffers trauma from an automobile accident during pregnancy.

Infections and Pregnancy

50.   Thrush in the newborn is directly related to contact in the birth canal with which of the following organisms?

a.   *Candida albicans*

b.   *Neisseria gonorrhoeae*

c.   *Treponema pallidum*

d.   *Staphylococcus aureus*

51.   In order to protect her unborn child from toxoplasmosis, a pregnant woman should

a.   avoid contact with people known to have German measles.

b.   avoid eating inadequately cooked meat.

c.   avoid sexual relations with known carriers of the causative organism.

d.   be vaccinated against it early in her pregnancy.

52.   Exposure to rubella during the _____ trimester is the time of greatest risk for teratogenic effects in the fetus.

Ⓡeflections

Think about a woman you have cared for or someone you have known whose pregnancy was considered high risk. What impact did it have on the woman and her family? How well did they cope? What actions by health care providers were helpful or not helpful?

_____

_____

_____

_____

_____

_____

_____

_____

53.   **Memory Check:** Define the following abbreviations.

a. CID

b. CMV

c. DIC

d. DTR

e. PIH

f. STD

g. STI

h. TORCH

9 | Assessment of Fetal Well-Being

This chapter corresponds to Chapter 14 in the 4th edition of *Maternal-Newborn Nursing Care: The Nurse, the Family, and the Community*.

Ultrasound

1. List two advantages for the mother and fetus of using ultrasound for assessment.

   a.

   b.

2. Identify at least six uses of ultrasound during early and late pregnancy.

Early Pregnancy (to 24 weeks)	Late Pregnancy (over 36 weeks)
a.	
b.	
c.	
d.	
e.	
f.	

3. Mrs Terrel Jackson is having an ultrasound examination. She asks, "Is it safe for my baby?" What will you say?

4. Hazel Applegate, G3 P1, is in her 23rd week of pregnancy. Her last normal menstrual period began 5½ months ago, but she had some bleeding 4½ months ago. Your physical assessment provides the following data: The fundus is palpable at two fingerbreadths below the umbilicus; the fetal heart rate (FHR) is 140. Hazel states that she has not felt quickening. Based on this information, why do you think Hazel will have an ultrasound done?

5. Hazel asks you what is involved in having an ultrasound. How will you respond?

Maternal Assessment of Fetal Activity

6. Carla Lewis is pregnant for the first time. She asks you how to monitor her baby's movements.

   a. Write out your teaching plan. On a separate sheet of paper, devise a score sheet that she could use.

   b. She asks if there is anything she can do that might affect the number of movements. How will you answer?

Nonstress Testing

7. What is the function of a nonstress test (NST)?

8. Explain the procedure for performing an NST.

9. Fetal heart rate patterns in NSTs have three classifications. Describe what a fetal monitoring strip would show in each case. What further testing may be indicated?

    a. Reactive

    b. Nonreactive

    c. Unsatisfactory

10. What is the best test result? Why?

11. Label each section of Figure 9–1A and B as reactive, nonreactive, or unsatisfactory.

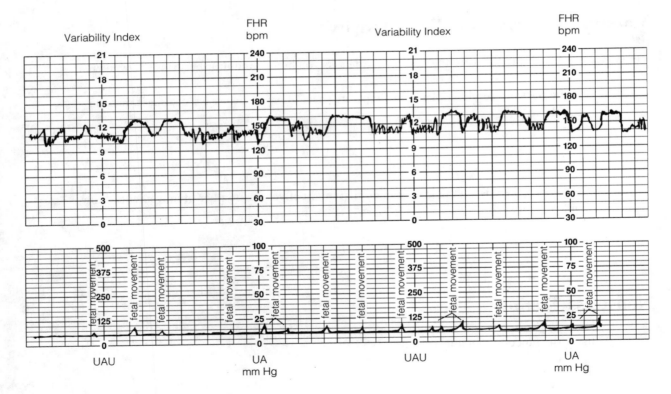

Figure 9–1A _____

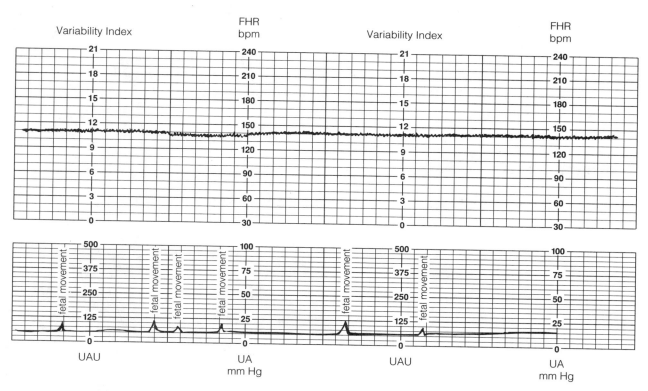

Figure 9–1B _____

12.   The NST can be modified by adding a fetal acoustic stimulation test (FAST). Describe how the FAST changes the basic NST.

Biophysical Profile

13.   A biophysical profile is completed to assess the fetus.

a.   Discuss the specific areas assessed in this test.

b.   How is it scored? What represents a "desirable" or "good" score?

c.   Describe the conditions in which it is most likely for a fetal biophysical profile to be done.

    d.   What does a decreased amniotic fluid volume mean?

    e.   Mr Kaplan calls the birth center and says, "My wife is to have a fetal biophysical profile tomorrow. What is it?" Write out how you will describe the assessment test to him.

Contraction Stress Testing

14.   List six indications for doing a contraction stress test (CST). Describe the physiologic rationale behind each indication.

    a.

    b.

    c.

    d.

    e.

    f.

15.   List three *contraindications* for the CST. Describe the physiologic rationale behind each.

16.   Describe the procedure for the breast self-stimulation test (BSST). (Also called nipple self-stimulation contraction stress test [NSCST].)

17.   Explain the major differences between BSST and CST with intravenous oxytocin (sometimes called oxytocin challenge test).

Match the CST results with their corresponding definitions.

18.   _____ Positive   a.   Late decelerations occur with 50% or more of the uterine contractions.

19.   _____ Negative   b.   No late decelerations occur with a minimum of three uterine contractions (lasting 40–60 seconds) in a 10-minute window.

20.   a.   Label the CST tracing in Figure 9–2 as positive or negative.

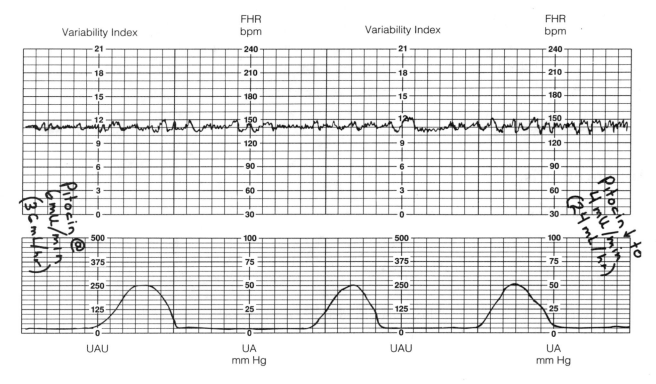

Figure 9–2 _____

b.   What factors led you to this conclusion?

21.   On the next tracing (Figure 9–3), draw your own test results. Use different colored ink so the tracings will stand out.

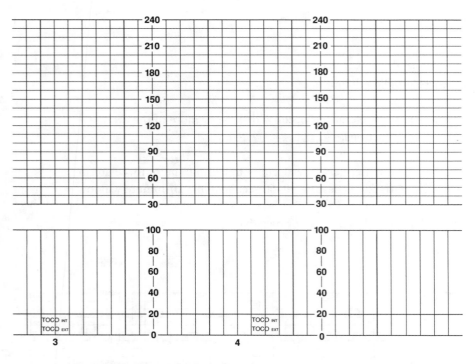

Figure 9–3

Amniocentesis

22.   What is the purpose of amniocentesis?

23.   What method may be used to locate the placenta prior to amniocentesis?

24.   List three nursing interventions necessary during amniocentesis.

ⓇReflections

Talk with a pregnant woman who is having prenatal testing done. What are her needs, concerns, and fears? Does she understand the reason for the test and what the test results mean? Does she know what to expect? What advice does she have for nurses who work in the antepartal testing situation?

_____

_____

_____

_____

_____

_____

---

25. List three complications associated with amniocentesis and the cause of each complication.

   a. _____   c. _____

   b. _____

26. Complete the chart on various tests that may be performed on amniotic fluid in the later portion of pregnancy.

Test	Purpose of Test	Normal Results	What Results Mean
(L/S) Lecithin/ Sphingomyelin Ratio			
Phosphatidylglycerol			
Creatinine			

27. **Critical Thinking in Practice:** The following action sequence is designed to help you think through clinical problems.

Holly Swit, a 37-year-old primipara, had an amniocentesis today. Holly calls the antepartal testing room 5 hours after her amniocentesis and says she is having contractions. Holly is at 38 weeks' gestation.

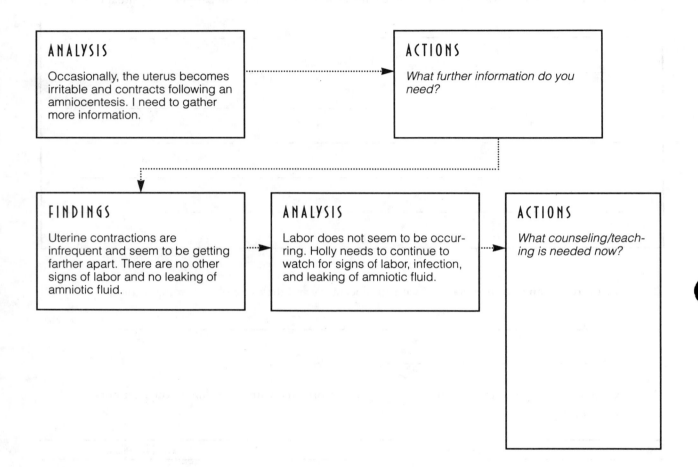

ANALYSIS

Occasionally, the uterus becomes irritable and contracts following an amniocentesis. I need to gather more information.

ACTIONS

What further information do you need?

FINDINGS

Uterine contractions are infrequent and seem to be getting farther apart. There are no other signs of labor and no leaking of amniotic fluid.

ANALYSIS

Labor does not seem to be occurring. Holly needs to continue to watch for signs of labor, infection, and leaking of amniotic fluid.

ACTIONS

What counseling/teaching is needed now?

28. **Critical Thinking Challenge:** The following situation has been developed to challenge your critical thinking. Read the situation and then answer "yes" or "no" to the question on page 95.

Your client, Amy Blankin, is a 15-year-old gravida 1 who is in her 35th week of pregnancy. An amniocentesis is done to assess fetal lung maturity. Test results indicate an L/S ratio of 2:1 and that prostaglandin (PG) is present.

Is fetal lung maturity indicated?

Yes _____   No _____

Explain your answer:

29. **Memory Check:** Define the following abbreviations.

a. AFV   i. HC

b. BBST   j. IUGR

c. BPP   k. L/S Ratio

d. CRL   l. NSCST

e. CST   m. NST

f. FAST   n. PG

g. FBM   o. US

h. FL   p. VST

10 | Birth: Processes and Stages

This chapter corresponds to Chapter 15 in the 4th edition of *Maternal-Newborn Nursing Care: The Nurse, the Family, and the Community.*

Maternal Pelvis

1. The majority of women have a gynecoid pelvis. The anthropoid pelvis is the second most common pelvic type. What characteristics of these pelves make them advantageous for birth?

2. The android and platypelloid pelves are unfavorable for vaginal birth. What unfavorable characteristics are present in each type?

3. Draw the shape of the pelvic inlet for each type of pelvis and mark the favorable characteristics with red pen to make them stand out.

4. The anterior posterior diameter of the pelvic inlet is estimated from manual measurement of the

  a. conjugate vera.

  b. diagonal conjugate. *(circled)*

  c. obstetric conjugate.

  d. intertuberishii.

5. The normal anterior-posterior diameter of the inlet needs to be at least

  a. 7 centimeters.

  b. 8 centimeters.

  c. 9 centimeters.

  d. 10 centimeters. *(circled)*

The Fetus

6. Label the parts of the fetal skull indicated in Figure 10–1.

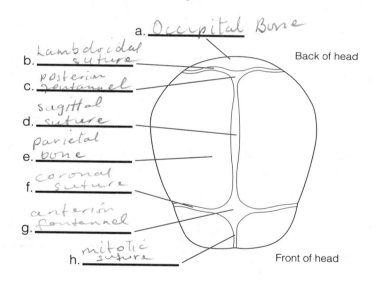

a. *Occipital Bone*

b. *Lambdoidal suture*

c. *posterior fontannel*

d. *sagittal suture*

e. *parietal bone*

f. *coronal suture*

g. *anterior fontannel*

h. *mitotic suture*

Back of head

Front of head

Figure 10–1   Superior view of the fetal skull.

7. Define *suture*. *The sutures of the fetal head are are membranous spaces between the cranial bones Intersection of sutures are called fontanneles*

Match the type of suture with its location.

8. ___C___ Mitotic (frontal) suture   a.   Between the parietal bones and the occipital bone

9. ___d___ Sagittal suture   b.   Between the parietal bones and the frontal bones

10. ___b___ Coronal suture   c.   Between the frontal bones

11. ___a___ Lambdoidal suture   d.   Between the parietal bones

12. Define *fontanelle*. Why are fontanelles important in the fetal skull?

13. Describe the location and characteristic size of the following:

   a.   Anterior fontanelle

   b.   Posterior fontanelle

14. Label the landmarks of the fetal skull indicated on Figure 10–2.

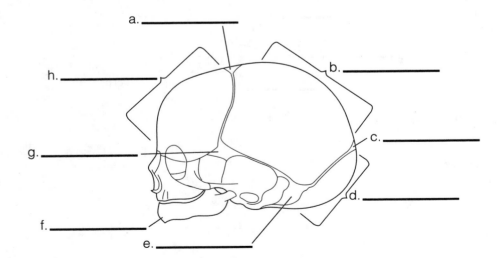

Figure 10–2   Lateral view of the fetal skull identifying the landmarks that have significance during birth.

15. Figure 10–3 depicts the anteroposterior and transverse diameters of the fetal head. Label each of the diameters and state the "norms" for an average size full-term newborn.

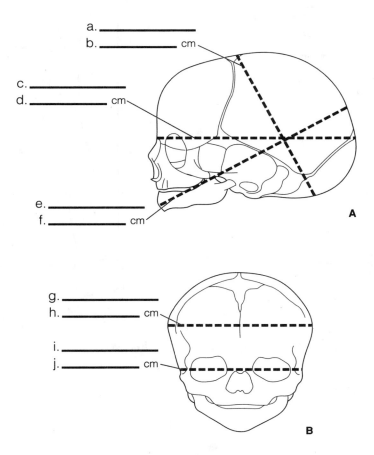

a. _____
b. _____ cm

c. _____
d. _____ cm

e. _____
f. _____ cm

A

g. _____
h. _____ cm

i. _____
j. _____ cm

B

Figure 10–3 **A.** Anteroposterior diameters of the fetal skull when the vertex of the fetus presents and the fetal head is flexed with the chin on the chest, the smallest anteroposterior diameter (suboccipitobregmatic diameter) enters the birth canal. **B.** Transverse diameters of the fetal skull.

Match the terms below with the correct definitions.

16. ___C___ Fetal attitude   a. Relationship of the cephalocaudal axis of the fetus to the cephalocaudal axis of the woman

17. ___A___ Fetal lie   b. Relationship of the landmark on the presenting fetal part to the anterior, posterior, or sides of the maternal pelvis

18. ___b___ Fetal position   c. Relationship of the fetal parts to one another

19.   Draw a fetus in a longitudinal lie and a transverse lie on Figure 10–4.

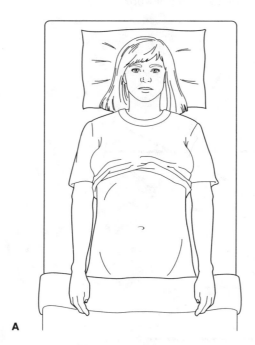   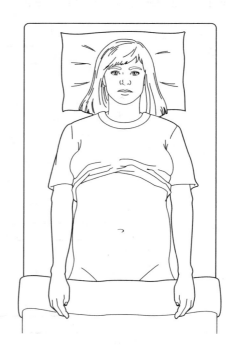

A   **B**

Figure 10–4   Fetal position.   **A.** Longitudinal lie.   **B.** Transverse lie.

20.   Define *fetal presentation*. determined by fetal lie and by the body part of the fetus that enters the mother pelvis first

21.   List the four types of cephalic presentation.

a. vertex   c. brow

b. military   d. face

22.   List and describe the three types of breech presentation. Explain how they are different.
       a. complete breech – fetal buttocks down against the cervix
       b. Frank breech – buttock down against the cervix fetal legs against abdomen and chest

c.

Label the fetal presentations and positions shown in Figure 10–5.

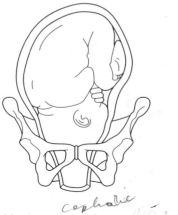
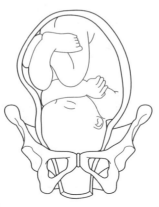
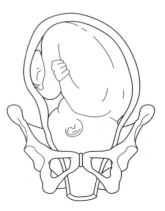

23. a. presentation ___cephalic___ _ROA_

    b. position ___ROA___

    c. presenting part ___Occiput___

24. a. presentation ___cephalic___

    b. position ___LOP___

    c. presenting part ___Occiput___

25. a. presentation ___C___

    b. position ___LOA___

    c. presenting part ___O___

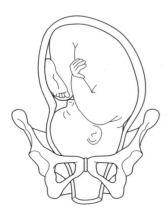
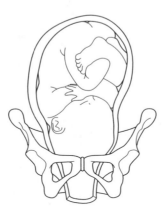
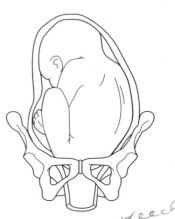

26. a. presentation ___C___

    b. position ___LOT___

    c. presenting part ___O___

27. a. presentation _____

    b. position ___ROT___

    c. presenting part ___O___

28. a. presentation ___breech___

    b. position ___LSA___

    c. presenting part ___Sacrum___

Figure 10–5 Categories of presentation. *(continued)*
SOURCE: Courtesy Ross Laboratories, Columbus, OH.

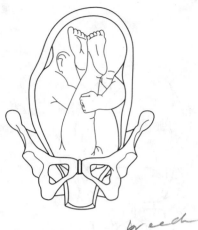

29. a. presentation _breech_

    b. position _RSA_

    c. presenting part _S_

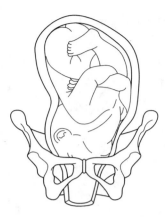

30. a. presentation _face_

    b. position _LMA_

    c. presenting part _mentum_

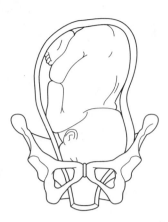

31. a. presentation _face_

    b. position _RMP_

    c. presenting part _Mentum_

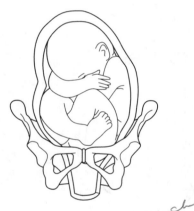

32. a. presentation _breech_

    b. position _LSP_

    c. presenting part _S_

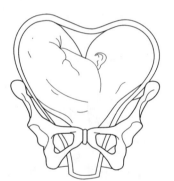

33. a. presentation _Transverse lie_

    b. position _LAPA_

    c. presenting part _Shoulder_

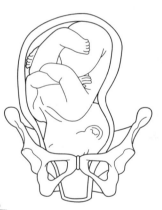

34. a. presentation _face_

    b. position _RMA_

    c. presenting part _mentum_

Figure 10–5   (continued)

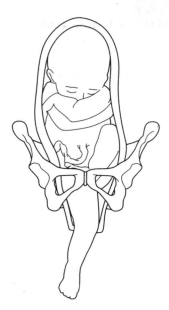

35. a. presentation _breech_
    b. position _single footling_
    c. presenting part _single footling_

Figure 10–5   *(continued)*

36.   List three methods that could be used to determine presentation and position.

a.

b.

c.

37.   Define *engagement*.

38.   What information does engagement provide about adequacy of the inlet, midpelvis, and outlet?

39.   Describe two methods used to determine engagement.

a.

b.

40. Devise two questions you could ask the expectant mother that would elicit information about symptoms indicative of engagement. Include your rationale.

    a.

    b.

41. Define *station*. How is station assessed?

42. Explain what a   1 station is.

43. Explain why the fetal presentation part may not descend.

Uterine Contractions

Match the term on the left to the correct definition on the right.

44. _____ Acme   a. The building up of the contraction

45. _____ Decrement   b. The letting up of the contraction

46. _____ Duration   c. The peak of the contraction

47. _____ Frequency   d. From the beginning of one to the beginning of the next contraction

48. _____ Increment   e. The time from the beginning to the end of one contraction

49. _____ Intensity   f. The strength of the contraction

50. Label each of the areas indicated in Figure 10–6.

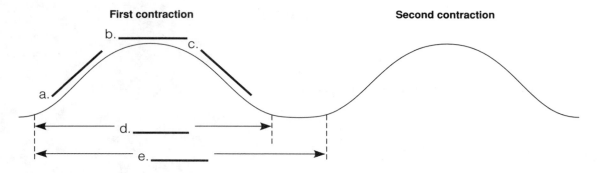

Figure 10–6 Characteristics of uterine contractions.

Psychosocial-Cultural Considerations

51.   Identify the factors that may affect a woman's psychologic response to labor.

52.   Describe how a woman's cultural background and preparation for labor might affect her psychologic status in labor.

Physiology of Labor

53.   Which of the following are considered premonitory signs of labor?

    a.   Bloody show, desire to bear down

    b.   Desire to bear down, increased vaginal secretions

    c.   Lightening, increased vaginal secretions

    d.   Rupture of membranes, elevated temperature

54.   There are various theories regarding the cause of labor onset. One possible cause involves

    a.   an increase in the amount of circulating progesterone.

    b.   a decrease in the amount of circulating estrogen.

    c.   production of endogenous oxytocin by the mother's pituitary gland.

    d.   inactivation of phospholipase A_2.

55.   The fetus adapts to the birth canal by undergoing some positional changes. Which of the following answers best describes the correct sequence?

    a.   Descent and flexion, extension, internal rotation, external rotation

    b.   Extension, descent and flexion, internal rotation, external rotation

    c.   Internal rotation, descent and flexion, extension, external rotation

    d.   Descent and flexion, internal rotation, extension, external rotation

56.   Labor and birth are divided into four stages, each with a definite beginning and ending. Complete the following chart:

Stage	Begins	Ends
First		
Second		
Third		
Fourth		

57.   The first stage of labor is divided into which three phases?

a.

b.

c.

Case Study: Read the scenario below, then answer questions 58–60 on page 107.

Sara Reed, a primigravida, is admitted to the birthing center. Sara states that she has been having contractions for 4 hours and her water broke just a little while ago. She is excited that she is in labor. An admission assessment reveals that the fetal heart rate is 140; contraction frequency is every 4–5 minutes, duration 40 seconds, intensity mild to moderate. Her cervix is 3 cm dilated and 50% effaced; fetal presentation is vertex, fetal station is −2, and the Nitrazine test tape is positive for amniotic fluid.

58.   What stage and phase of labor is Sara in?

59.   a.   How much dilatation would you expect every hour for Sara?

      b.   How would this be different if Sara was a multigravida?

60.   What will contractions probably be like when Sara is in the transition phase?

Reflections

Frequently the experience of labor is much different from the "norms" that textbooks address because each individual is different. What was your labor or the labor of a client like? Did it match the characteristics that you are learning about now? How was it different?

_____

_____

_____

_____

_____

_____

_____

61.   Discuss the physiologic causes of pain during labor and birth.

62.   Identify key factors that affect the woman's response to pain.

63.   **Memory Check:** Define the following abbreviations.

a.   LADA

b.   LADP

c.   LMA

d.   LMP

e.   LMT

f.   LOA

g.   LOP

h.   LOT

i.   LSA

j.   LSP

k.   LST

l.   RMA

m.   RMP

n.   RMT

o.   ROA

p.   ROM

q.   ROP

r.   ROT

s.   RSA

t.   RSP

u.   RST

11

Nursing Assessment and Care of the Intrapartal Family

This chapter corresponds to Chapter 16 in the 4th edition of *Maternal-Newborn Nursing Care: The Nurse, the Family, and the Community.*

Initial Assessment and Admission

1.   The following questionnaire is similar to many that are used when a woman is admitted to the labor and birth unit. Have a friend or family member act as a client and role-play a situation in which you, as the labor and birth nurse, complete the interview. (Note: this questionnaire focuses primarily on baseline information and does not include information that would require physical assessment.)

Admission date _____ Time _____ Admitting nurse _____

Patient name _____ Age _____

EDB _____ LMP _____ Length of gestation by dates _____

Attending MD/CNM _____ Pediatrician _____

Gravida _____ Para _____ Ab _____ Living children _____

Onset of labor: Spontaneous _____ Induced _____ Time _____ Bleeding _____

Membrane status: Intact _____ Ruptured _____ Time _____

Blood type _____ Rh _____ Serology _____ Date of serology of testing _____

Persons for maternal support during birth _____

Prenatal education classes: Yes _____ No _____ Type _____

Birthing requests: Feeding method: Breast _____ Bottle _____ Glucose water _____

Prep: Yes _____ No _____ Enema: Yes _____ No _____ Ambulation: Yes _____ No _____

Shower: Yes _____ No _____ Jacuzzi: Yes _____ No _____ Fetal monitor: Yes _____ No _____

Choices of labor position _____ Birthing position _____

→

Medication during labor: Yes _____ No _____   Regional block: Yes _____ No _____

Birth requests _____

Other _____

Prepregnancy weight _____ Present weight _____ Weight gain _____

Allergy: Medications _____ Foods _____ Substances _____

Time of last food intake _____ Type _____ Fluids _____

Medical problems prior to pregnancy _____

Problems with last pregnancy _____

Problems with this pregnancy _____

2. Allison Scott is admitted to the birthing center accompanied by her husband, Dave. She is in early labor. During your initial interview, you discover that she is a primigravida and that her expected date of birth (EDB) is today. She has not attended prenatal classes. What four observations will you make while assessing her contractions?

   a.

   b.

   c.

   d.

3. Why do you use your fingertips instead of the palm of your hand to palpate contractions?

4. What would you expect Allison's contractions to be like if she is in the latent phase?

5. The charge nurse records Allison's contractions as every 5 minutes, lasting 30 seconds, and of mild intensity.

   a. What is the frequency? _____

   b. What is the duration? _____

   c. What is the intensity? _____

6.   Dave hands you a piece of paper with a recording of contractions prior to admission. The paper shows:

CONTRACTION BEGINS	CONTRACTION ENDS
0500:00	0500:40
0505:00	0505:40
0508:00	0508:45
0511:00	0511:45

a.   What is the frequency of the contractions? _____

b.   What is the duration of the contractions? _____

7.   What differences would you perceive when palpating mild, moderate, and strong (intense) contractions?

8.   You will use a hand-held Doppler to assess fetal heart rate (FHR).

a.   Describe the method you will use to locate the FHR.

b.   After locating the fetal heartbeat and just before counting the FHR, you check Allison's radial pulse. Explain the rationale for this.

c.   How long should you listen to the FHR? At what times will it be important to assess the FHR?

9.   As part of your assessment, you perform Leopold's maneuvers on Allison. How should she be positioned?

10. When you do Leopold's maneuvers, you feel a firm, rounded object in the uterine fundus; a smooth surface along the right side of the uterus (mother's right side); a surface that feels more nodular on the left side of the uterus; and a body part that is rounded and even more firm just above the symphysis.

   a. The fetal presentation is _____.

   b. The fetal position is _____.

11. Explain why membrane status should be ascertained before a vaginal examination is done.

12. What effect do intact membranes have on labor progress?

13. Explain the implications of ruptured membranes for the mother and fetus.

14. Why do you need to know the exact time that the membranes rupture?

15. Explain why the FHR is assessed immediately after the membranes have ruptured.

16. Allison says she doesn't think she wants her membranes ruptured artificially, but she's not sure. She asks, "What do you think I should do?" Write out your answer. Remember, because you want to help her be an informed consumer, your answer needs to include assessment of Allison's knowledge and understanding, an overview of the purpose of amniotomy, advantages, disadvantages, and any known alternatives to the amniotomy.

17. To practice your role as client advocate, imagine you have just carefully explained an amniotomy to a woman, and she decides she doesn't want it done. The physician calls in and says, "I'm on my way to the birthing unit to see Mrs X. I'm planning to do an amniotomy if all is going well." What will your response be?

18. While examining Mrs X, the physician says, "Hand me an amnihook so I can rupture these membranes." Mrs X quickly looks to you, shaking her head from side to side. What will you say?

19. Allison states that she is losing some clear fluid from her vagina when she coughs. You note that the Nitrazine test tape does not change color.

   a. Are the membranes intact or ruptured?

   b. What do you think the source of the clear fluid is?

20. You do a vaginal examination on Allison.

   a. List the information that can be ascertained by performing a vaginal examination.

   b. How do you position Allison for the vaginal examination? What will you do to protect her privacy?

21. During the vaginal examination, you find that you can place two fingers side by side in Allison's cervix. You can feel a firm surface against the cervix and a softer triangular shape in the upper right position (between 12 and 3 on a clock). You also note a small amount of bloody show.

   a. What is the cervical dilatation?

   b. What is the presentation?

   c. What is the position?

   d. What causes the bloody show?

22.   The obstetrician has ordered a "miniprep" and a Fleet's enema for Allison if she wants them.

   a.   Allison does not understand what a "miniprep" is. What nursing actions will you take to allow her to participate in an informed way?

   b.   What are three effects an enema may have on labor and birth?

   c.   If an enema is given, what safety factors should you consider when Allison is ready to expel the enema?

Breathing Techniques

23.   Choose a breathing technique commonly used in your area. Now, select a friend and teach them the breathing pattern you chose. Write out a description or draw the breathing pattern so you will be ready for your clinical experience.

24.   What can you do to help Dave during the birth process? How can you assist him in supporting Allison? Describe support and comfort measures you can teach him or that you can provide if needed.

Fetal Monitoring

The physician has recommended fetal monitoring for a short time. After the reason for it is explained, Allison agrees to having a monitor placed on her.

25.   Define the following terms used with fetal monitoring:

   a.   Fetal baseline

   b.   Fetal tachycardia

   c.   Fetal bradycardia

   d.   Baseline variability

   e.   Early deceleration

   f.   Late deceleration

   g.   Variable deceleration

26.   Spell out the following abbreviations used in fetal monitoring:

   a.   EFM

   b.   FHR

   c.   UA

   d.   UPI

   e.   HC

   f.   CC

27.   The normal fetal heart rate is (a) _____ to (b) _____ bpm, short-term variability is

   (c) _____, long-term variability is (d) _____, there are accelerations with fetal

   movement, and there are (e) _____ late or variable decelerations.

28. List five possible causes of fetal tachycardia.

    a.

    b.

    c.

    d.

    e.

29. List three possible causes of fetal bradycardia.

    a.

    b.

    c.

30. List three possible causes of changes in baseline variability.

    a.

    b.

    c.

31. Explain the causes and the physiologic rationale for the following:

    a. Early deceleration

    b. Late deceleration

    c. Variable deceleration

34. Evaluate the fetal monitoring strip (Figure 11–3).

   a. Contraction frequency _____

   b. Contraction duration _____

   Type of FHR pattern (check one of the following):

   _____ early decelerations

   _____ late decelerations

   _____ variable decelerations

   Circle each deceleration you find.

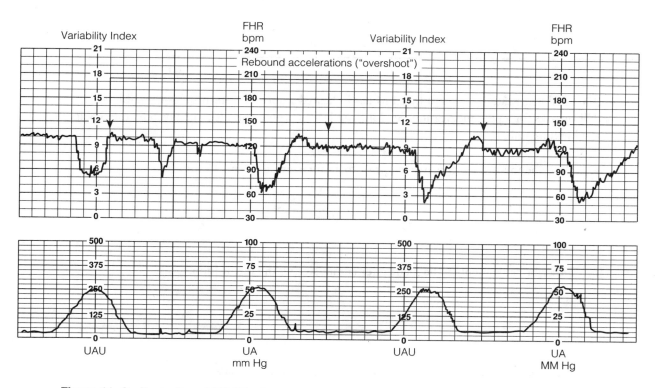

Figure 11–3 Evaluation of EFM Tracing.

35.   Identify the immediate nursing actions and physiologic rationale for the following
FHR problems:

FHR Problem	Nursing Actions	Physiologic Rationale
Late decelerations		
Variable decelerations		

36.   The fetal heart rate assessment by EFM has indicated a normal pattern. At 5–6 cm dilatation,
Allison asks for a pain medication. Stadol 1 mg IVP is ordered and is to be given by the RN in
the birthing unit.

    a.   Describe the assessments needed prior to administering the medication.

    b.   Describe assessments to be made after administering the medication.

    c.   List at least two indications that the medication is exerting the expected effect.

37.   Allison reaches 8 cm and becomes restless and impatient. What phase of labor is she in?

Assessment and Support During Labor

38.   Allison begins to indicate many signs of discomfort and anxiety. Her previous methods to increase relaxation are no longer effective. Based on your assessment, you select the nursing diagnosis Pain related to anxiety and difficulty maintaining relaxation. Identify at least four nursing interventions you think are important. Explain the physiologic rationale for each intervention.

     a.   **Nursing Intervention**   **Physiologic Rationale**

     b.   Identify two anticipated outcomes or two signs that would indicate your interventions have been effective.

39.   Allison complains of tingling and numbness in her hands and feet.

     a.   What is the cause?

     b.   List nursing interventions to assist Allison.

     c.   Identify findings that indicate your interventions have been effective.

40.   Allison reaches complete dilatation.

      a. Complete dilatation is _____ cm.

      b. What stage of labor is Allison in?

41.   List signs that indicate birth is imminent.

42.   You prepare the birthing room for the birth. Describe the maternal positions that may be used during labor and birth. Identify the advantages and disadvantages of each and determine one situation in which you might suggest the use of that particular position.

43.   How often will you assess blood pressure and FHR in the second stage?

44.   Explain the support and comfort measures you or Dave can use to help Allison feel more comfortable as birth approaches.

Episiotomy

45.   The physician tells Allison that an episiotomy is needed. Describe indications for an episiotomy.

46.   In Figure 11–4, draw a midline, left mediolateral, and right mediolateral episiotomy.

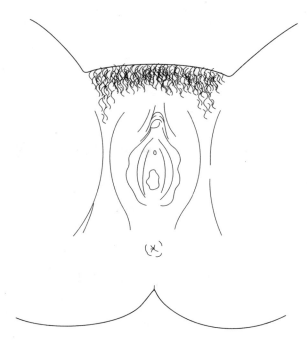

Figure 11–4

47.   Complete the following chart regarding differences between a midline episiotomy and medio-lateral episiotomy.

Characteristic	Midline Episiotomy	Mediolateral Episiotomy
Indication		
Healing		
Discomfort after birth		

48. Discuss prenatal measures and interventions during labor and birth that may decrease the need for an episiotomy.

Birth

49. As the baby's head begins to emerge, the obstetrician/certified nurse-midwife supports it with their hand. Explain the rationale for this.

50. Why are the baby's nose and mouth suctioned as soon as the head has emerged?

Apgar Score

51. A baby boy is born. Your first assessment of him provides the following information:
    Heart rate 124
    Respirations 24 and irregular
    Flexion and movement of all extremities
    Vigorous crying when suctioned with the bulb syringe
    Pink body with some acrocyanosis

	0	1	2
Heart rate	Absent	Slow (below 100)	Above 100
Respiratory effort	Absent	Slow, irregular	Good crying
Muscle tone	Flaccid	Some flexion of extremities	Active motion
Reflex irritability	None	Grimace	Vigorous cry
Color	Pale, blue	Body pink, extremities blue	Completely pink

Fig 11–5 Sample Apgar scoring sheet. (Modified from Apgar V: The newborn [Apgar] scoring system: Reflection and advice. *Pediatr Clin N Am* [Aug] 1966; 13:645)

    a.   Record the preceding assessments on the Apgar scoring sheet (Figure 11–5).

    b.   What is the total Apgar score? _____

    c.   Apgar scores are assessed at _____ minutes and _____ minutes following birth.

52.   The most crucial of the Apgar assessments are the heart rate and respiration. If the baby has a pink body, what do you know about the baby's heartbeat and respiration?

Nursing Care Following Birth

53.   List the methods that may be used to provide warmth to the newborn in the birthing room.

54.   Why should the newborn be dried thoroughly as soon after birth as possible?

55.   Allison places her newborn on her chest with skin-to-skin contact to maintain warmth. In some birth settings the newborn may be placed under a radiant heater. Explain how the radiant heater works.

56.   As the nurse, you assess the number of vessels on the umbilical cord.

    a.   Why is this important?

    b.   How many vessels should there be?

57.   List two methods of assuring correct identification of the newborn after birth.

a.

b.

58.   What positions may the baby be placed in to facilitate drainage of the respiratory tract?

59.   What complication may result from vigorous, frequent oral suctioning?

60.   List the areas that will be checked during a brief physical assessment of the newborn in the first few minutes after birth.

61.   Describe ways you can facilitate attachment immediately after birth.

62.   List specific maternal behaviors that would indicate Allison is beginning to establish attachment.

Delivery of the Placenta

63.   List four signs that indicate separation of the placenta.

   a.

   b.

   c.

   d.

64.   Describe differences between a Schultze and a Duncan expulsion of the placenta.

   a.   Method of separation from the uterine wall

   b.   Appearance of placenta at the moment of exit from the vagina

65.   Identify the complications that may be associated with a Duncan placenta.

66.   List three assessments of the expelled placenta that need to be made.

Nursing Care in the Third Stage

67.   The obstetrician orders 10 units of Pitocin given IVP after expulsion of the placenta.

   a.   Explain the rationale for administration of an oxytocic medication following expulsion of the placenta.

   b.   Identify the most important nursing interventions when administering Pitocin.

68.   You need to record the length of each stage on Allison's birth record, based on the following information:

Contractions began at 0800
Complete dilatation at 1600
Delivered male infant at 1710
Delivered placenta at 1725

a. First stage   _____

b. Second stage   _____

c. Third stage   _____

d. Fourth stage   _____

69.   How does the length of each of Allison's stages compare with "norms" for primigravidas?

Nursing Care in the Fourth Stage

Allison begins her recovery period after birth. For each of the critical nursing assessments listed, indicate the expected normal findings. Circle the correct answer.

70.   Blood pressure and pulse

a.   same as in labor

b.   elevated

c.   at prepregnant level

71.   Uterine fundus height

a.   above umbilicus

b.   at umbilicus

c.   below umbilicus

85. How do each of the following factors influence the perception of pain in the laboring woman?

   a. Cultural background

   b. Fatigue

   c. Anxiety

   d. Previous experience

86. The nurse completes pertinent assessments of the mother, the baby, and the labor prior to administering analgesics during labor. For each of the following, indicate findings that should be present prior to administration of the analgesic.

   a. Maternal assessment

   b. Fetal assessment

   c. Labor assessment

87. Barbara Adams, gravida 1 para 0, is in the active phase of labor. Contractions are every 3 minutes, lasting 50 seconds, and are moderate. She is 7 cm dilated, 75% effaced, and at 0 station. Her membranes are intact, and the FHR is 140. With each contraction, Barbara cries out and thrashes in the bed. Her restlessness continues between contractions. She repeatedly changes positions and rolls her head from side to side. Her blood pressure and pulse rate have increased over the past 2 hours. The physician has ordered 75 mg of meperidine and 25 mg of promethazine given intramuscularly when needed for pain.

   a. In the above statement, circle all the findings that indicate it would be safe to administer the ordered medication. (Note: see answer to question 86 to assist you if you are having difficulty.)

   b. Identify the three most important nursing considerations regarding administration of medication.

c. If all you have is a 100 mg/1 mL ampule of Demerol, how much will you draw up in your syringe?

d. Identify the landmarks you would use to administer the medication in the:

(1) dorsogluteal site.

(2) ventrogluteal site.

88. If Barbara continues to experience discomfort and needs additional pain relief, what types of regional anesthesia might be given?

a. In active labor:

b. In second stage labor:

89. For which of the following women would administration of analgesia seem most appropriate?

a. 3 cm, with contractions every 4 to 5 minutes, lasting 30 seconds, and of mild intensity

b. 5 cm, with contractions every 3 minutes, lasting 50 seconds, and of moderate to strong intensity; FHR 140 with good variability; woman relaxing well and breathing with contractions

c. 7 cm, with contractions every 3 minutes, lasting 50 seconds, and of moderate to strong intensity; FHR 140 with minimal variability and occasional late deceleration

d. 7 cm, with contractions every 3 minutes, lasting 50 seconds, and of moderate to strong intensity; FHR 140 with good variability; woman tense and unable to relax between contractions

90. **Critical Thinking in Practice:** The following action sequence is designed to help you think through clinical problems. Read the sequence below, then fill in the appropriate boxes in the flowchart on page 133.

You are the nurse in the birthing area. Carolyn Morse, a 25-year-old gravida 2 para 1, has been laboring for the past 6 hours. Suddenly you hear a low groan from her room, and then Carolyn begins to shout, "The baby is coming!" You rush to her room.

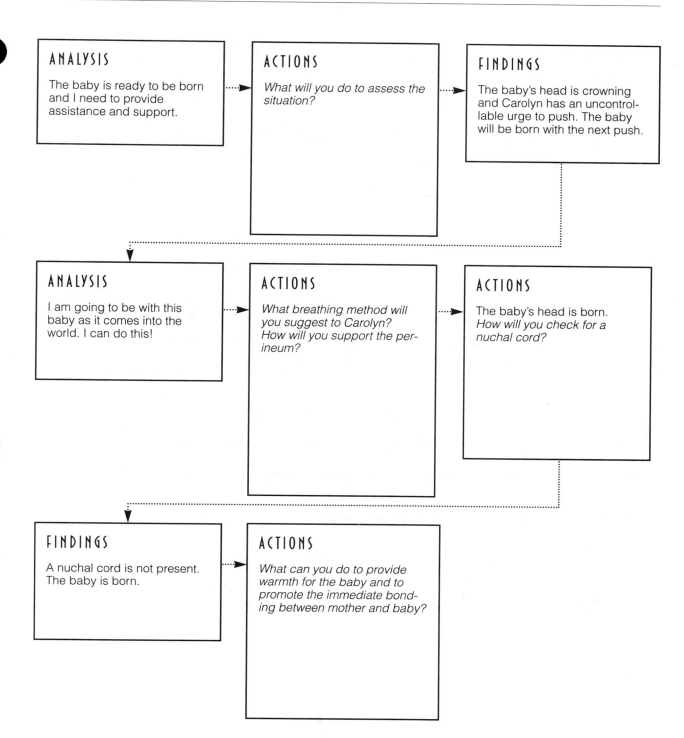

ANALYSIS

The baby is ready to be born and I need to provide assistance and support.

ACTIONS

What will you do to assess the situation?

FINDINGS

The baby's head is crowning and Carolyn has an uncontrollable urge to push. The baby will be born with the next push.

ANALYSIS

I am going to be with this baby as it comes into the world. I can do this!

ACTIONS

What breathing method will you suggest to Carolyn? How will you support the perineum?

ACTIONS

The baby's head is born. *How will you check for a nuchal cord?*

FINDINGS

A nuchal cord is not present. The baby is born.

ACTIONS

What can you do to provide warmth for the baby and to promote the immediate bonding between mother and baby?

Ⓡeflections

Describe the first birth that you were able to attend as a student nurse. What support measures were used? Did the expectant woman have a support person? How was the newborn welcomed into the world by those present? What were your feelings?

_____

_____

_____

_____

_____

_____

_____

_____

91.   **Memory Check:** Define the following abbreviations.

a. Ab   g. HC

b. EDB   h. LMP

c. EFM   i. Rh

d. Dec   j. ROM

e. epis   k. VBAC

f. FHR

12 | Complications of the Intrapartal Period

This chapter corresponds to Chapters 19 and 20 in the 4th edition of *Maternal-Newborn Nursing Care: The Nurse, the Family, and the Community.*

Anxiety Regarding Labor and Birth

1. Anxiety may have untoward effects on the laboring woman and her baby. Explain the possible effects of increased anxiety and fear on the birth process.

2. Describe the signs and symptoms you might observe when a woman is experiencing fear and anxiety.

3. Identify at least one nursing diagnosis that would be important in decreasing a woman's anxiety and fear.

Failure to Progress

4.   Compare the effects of hypertonic and hypotonic labor on the woman and her baby.

5.   Discuss the recommended treatment for hypotonic labor and failure to progress.

Precipitous Labor and Birth

6.   Define *precipitous labor.*

7.   Discuss the medical treatment that may be suggested for subsequent births when a woman has had a precipitous labor and birth.

Postterm Pregnancy

Laura Collins, a 21-year-old primipara, is pregnant with her first child. Laura's last menstrual period (LMP) was September 8.

8.   Her expected date of birth (EDB) is:

9.   On what date would her pregnancy become postterm?

10. Laura does have a postterm pregnancy. Why will the fetus be at increased risk of having a variable deceleration pattern? What other problems may occur during labor and birth?

Amnioinfusion

11. Grace Yoo is also experiencing postterm pregnancy. Her CNM orders a biophysical profile to assess the fetus. The BPP is 6 with decreased amniotic fluid and a nonreactive nonstress test. The FHR exhibits numerous variable decelerations. The decision is made to treat the oligohydramnios and variable decelerations by doing an amnioinfusion and then inducing labor. What is an amnioinfusion and how do you know whether it is achieving the desired effect?

12. What other nursing interventions might you use to assist in relieving variable decelerations?

13. Why is the fetus at risk for meconium aspiration when oligohydramnios is present?

Induction of Labor

14.   List two indications for induction of labor. Explain why the induction may need to be done.

    a.

    b.

15.   Patricia Gomez is scheduled for induction of labor. She is at 40 weeks' gestation. Prior to induction, a CST is obtained and the results are positive. Identify any contraindications present in the above example.

16.   List additional factors that contraindicate induction.

TABLE 12-1 Prelabor status evaluation scoring (Bishop) system

| Factor | Assigned value | | | |
	0	**1**	**2**	**3**
Cervical dilatation	Closed	1–2 cm	3–4 cm	5 cm or more
Cervical effacement	0%–30%	40%–50%	60%–70%	80% or more
Fetal station	−3	−2	−1,0	+1 or lower
Cervical consistency	Firm	Moderate	Soft	
Cervical position	Posterior	Midposition	Anterior	

Modified from Bishop EH: Pelvic scoring for elective induction. *Obstet Gynecol* 1964; 24:266.

17.   Explain the Bishop score (see Table 12–1). What implications would the following scores have on anticipated induction success?

    a.   Score of 3

    b.   Score of 9

18.   Amanda White is admitted for an induction. She is gravida 2 para 1 and at 42 weeks' gestation. Her membranes are intact. Amanda's obstetrician orders a continuous fetal monitor with a 15-minute baseline, followed by an intravenous induction of 10 units Pitocin in 1000 mL 5% dextrose in lactated Ringer's. The Pitocin is to be started at 1 mU (milliunit)/min by IV infusion pump. How many milliliters per hour will be needed to infuse 1 mU/min?

19.   Five percent dextrose in water is not routinely used for Pitocin induction because of the risk of water intoxication. Describe the signs of water intoxication.

20.   Describe the physical assessments and the findings that indicate Amanda's infusion rate can be advanced.

21.   Identify the problems that might occur in response to the Pitocin induction.

22.   After the induction has been in process for 2 hours, you palpate strong contractions and note the following information on the fetal monitoring strip (see Figure 12–1) on page 140.

   a.   FHR baseline is _____ bpm

   b.   STV is present _____ absent _____

   c.   LTV is _____

   d.   Accelerations are present. Yes _____ No _____

   e.   Contraction frequency is _____

   f.   Contraction duration is _____

   g.   Based on your assessment, should the IV Pitocin infusion rate be advanced? Explain your decision.

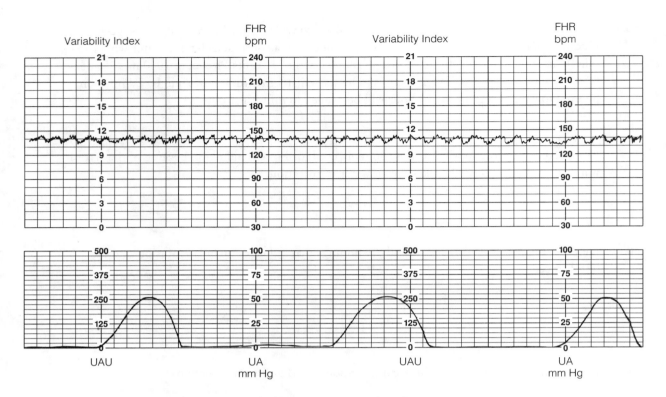

Figure 12–1   Fetal heart tracings. Six small spaces equal 1 minute.

23.   After an additional 1 hour of induction, you observe the fetal monitoring strip (see Figure 12–2) on page 141. What should you do?

a.   What immediate nursing actions need to be taken?

b.   What information from the strip did you use to determine your nursing actions?

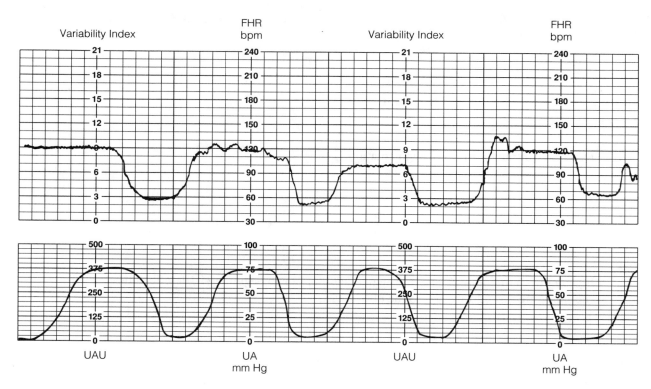

Figure 12–2   Fetal monitoring strip. 6 small spaces equal 1 minute.

24.   The obstetrician decides to rupture Amanda's membranes.

    a.   Why might this be done?

    b.   What two assessments should be made immediately after the membranes are ruptured?

25.   Explain the significance of the following characteristics of amniotic fluid:

    a.   Greenish color

    b.   Reddish color

    c.   Foul odor

26. Intravenous Pitocin may be used for augmentation of labor. Explain the differences between induction of labor and augmentation of labor.

27. Describe contraindications to augmentation.

28. If you note contraindications to the augmentation prior to beginning it, describe how you will communicate this information to the obstetrician.

Fetal Malposition

Match the fetal malposition on the left with the descriptions on the right. More than one description may be used for each fetal malposition.

29. _____ Occiput posterior position

30. _____ Face presentation

31. _____ Brow presentation

32. _____ Transverse lie

a. Largest anteroposterior of the fetal head presents to the maternal pelvis.

b. The shoulder or acromion process is the presenting part.

c. A cesarean birth must be done.

d. The laboring woman experiences severe backache.

e. Pelvic rocking may convert the OP to OA.

f. The anteroposterior diameter of the fetal head is small, but the baby is at great risk during vaginal birth.

g. If the mentum is posterior, a cesarean is the method of birth.

33. Label each type of breech and the position of each on Figure 12–3.

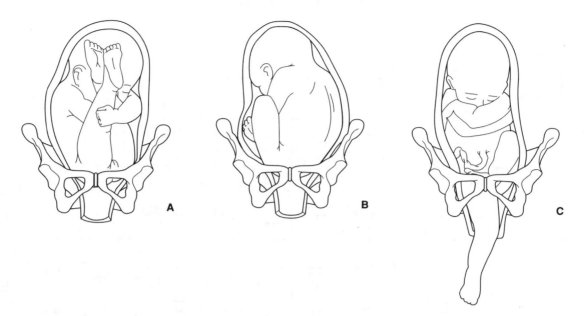

Figure 12–3 Types of breech.

a. _____   b. _____   c. _____

34. Breech presentation carries an increased risk of prolapse of the umbilical cord. Draw a prolapsed cord in Figure 12–3c. Use a colored pen or pencil so it will stand out.

35. Prolapse of the cord causes pressure on the umbilical cord.

a. Explain the fetal implications of a prolapsed cord.

b. Describe what you would feel while performing a sterile vaginal exam, and what your immediate interventions must be.

c.   On Figure 12–4, draw the type of deceleration pattern that may occur with a prolapsed cord. First draw uterine contractions with a frequency of 3 minutes.

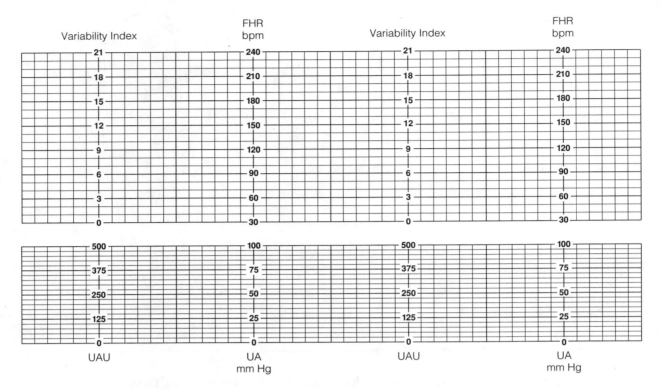

Figure 12–4

External Version

36.   At 38 weeks' gestation, an external version may be done to convert a breech presentation into a cephalic presentation.

a.   Identify the prerequisites for a version and include rationale.

b.   Discuss nursing interventions before, during, and after the version.

c.   Why would an Rh-negative woman need to receive RhoGAM?

d.   Write out the pertinent points you need to cover in discharge teaching.

Multiple Pregnancy

37.   Lisa Rote is in her second pregnancy. List two signs and symptoms that may indicate the presence of twins.

a.

b.

38.   Identify three implications of the multiple pregnancy for Lisa.

a.

b.

c.

39.   Discuss the treatment that will be suggested for Lisa during her pregnancy.

40.   Discuss the implications of the multiple pregnancy for the fetuses during labor and birth.

41.   During labor, both fetuses will be monitored by electronic fetal monitoring. If one fetus begins to demonstrate problems with fetal heart rate (FHR), what will need to occur?

42.   List three signs and symptoms that would indicate fetal distress.

       a.

       b.

       c.

43.   The major maternal complication that may occur following birth of twins is (a) _____ .
       This occurs because (b) _____ .

Fetal Distress: Meconium-Stained Amniotic Fluid

44.   Meleah Stone, gravida 3 para 2, is admitted with contractions every 2 minutes, lasting 60 seconds and of strong intensity. Her membranes ruptured spontaneously 2 hours ago, and Meleah reports the fluid has been "greenish." She is breathing well with contractions and denies any discomfort. When assessing FHR, you located it above the umbilicus, at 140 beats per minute and regular. What would you suspect?

45.   Explain the possible reasons for the presence of greenish amniotic fluid. What special measures will need to be taken for the newborn immediately after birth due to the presence of the green-stained fluid?

Intrauterine Fetal Death

46.   Anna Marinara, a 19-year-old primipara, calls the birthing unit and tells you she hasn't felt her baby move for two days.

    a.   When she arrives, you admit her and listen for the FHR. You don't hear anything with the ultrasound Doppler. She says, "Did you hear my baby? Is she alive?" What will you say?

    b.   What testing will you be able to anticipate for her?

47.   Describe nursing care that will be important for Anna and her partner.

Placental Problems

48.   Define *abruptio placentae*. What are the different types?

49.   Define *placenta previa*. What are the different types?

Match the placental problems on the left with the descriptions on the right. Descriptions may be used more than once.

50. _____ Abruptio placenta (marginal)   a.   Bright red bleeding without pain

51. _____ Abruptio placenta (central)   b.   Dark red bleeding, may be associated with pain

52. _____ Placenta previa (complete)   c.   Uterine tenderness and irritability

                                                d.   Normal uterine tone

                                                e.   Increased resting tone between contractions

                                                f.   Increased risk of DIC

53. Maria Thomas is admitted at 38 weeks' gestation with abruptio placentae. She is at increased risk for DIC and HELLP. Why are these complications more likely to develop?

54. Dortha Haney, gravida 3 para 1, is admitted with moderate vaginal bleeding. She is at 39 weeks' gestation. She states that she is not having contractions but that she has had episodes of vaginal bleeding since the 20th week. An ultrasound reading demonstrated a marginal placenta previa. The FHR is 140. You know that a vaginal examination is usually done on admission to assess cervical dilatation. Will you do a vaginal examination now? Give the rationale for your answer.

Amniotic Fluid Embolism

55. Mrs Carey is a 28-year-old G2 P1 in active labor. She suddenly begins exhibiting signs and symptoms of amniotic fluid embolus. What will you be seeing?

     a.   You know that amniotic fluid embolus is more likely in particular situations. Write out a possible history for Mrs Carey that includes factors associated with amniotic fluid embolism.

b.   Describe the medical treatment that must be initiated immediately for Mrs Carey.

Hydramnios

56.   Hydramnios occurs when there is more than _____ mL of amniotic fluid in the uterus.

57.   Polly Brooks is diagnosed as having hydramnios. List three physical changes this may cause and identify at least two self-care measures you could suggest.

58.   Identify three fetal problems associated with hydramnios and a method of identifying each problem.

    a.

    b.

    c.

59.   When Polly's membranes rupture, she will be at increased risk for abruptio placentae. Explain the reason for this.

Oligohydramnios

60.   Define *oligohydramnios*.

61.   Which fetal deceleration pattern are you more likely to see with oligohydramnios? Why?

62. Explain why oligohydramnios may be present when the fetus has a malformation or malfunction of the genitourinary system.

Cephalopelvic Disproportion

63. Mrs Gonzales has a diagonal conjugate of 10 cm and converging side walls, and the fetal BPD (biparietal diameter) is 10 cm. What implications does this have for her labor and birth?

64. What types of evaluation methods would you expect to be done when CPD (cephalopelvic disproportion) is suspected?

65. Explain the rationale for a "trial of labor" (TOL) for a woman with borderline pelvic measurements.

66. What progress would you expect in cervical dilatation if the dilatation pattern remained within normal limits?

67. What progress would you expect in fetal descent?

68. In what instances would a cesarean need to be done?

69. Give an example in which the woman might need a cesarean for one birth and not for subsequent ones.

Forceps-Assisted Birth

70. List three indications for the use of forceps to assist in vaginal birth.

     a.

     b.

     c.

71. Identify the criteria that should be met in order for the obstetrician to use forceps safely.

72. Define the following:

     a. Outlet forceps

     b. Low forceps

     c. Mid-forceps

73. Identify complications (maternal and fetal) that may be associated with forceps.

74.   Discuss the nursing interventions that are necessary during an outlet forceps–assisted birth. Include the teaching that should be done.

75.   The new parents you worked with last evening during a forceps-assisted birth stop you in the hall today and ask why their baby's face is bruised and swollen on one side. They ask if it will go away. What will you tell them?

Vacuum Extractor–Assisted Birth

76.   A vacuum extractor may be used instead of forceps.

    a.   Explain how this works.

    b.   Why might the baby have a "chignon"? Write out the important points to include in your parent teaching if the baby has a "chignon."

    c.   Describe the teaching that will be needed prior to the use of the vacuum extractor. (Include maternal and fetal information.)

Cesarean Birth

77.   Janel Thompson, a 24-year-old gravida 2 para 1, at 30 weeks' gestation, is admitted to the birthing area for a repeat cesarean. Her primary (first) cesarean was done as an emergency measure when she began bleeding heavily from a complete placenta previa. The L/S ratio is 2.5:1 and PG is present.

a.   Describe how you will do the abdominal perineal prep.

b.   Describe the procedure for inserting an indwelling bladder catheter. What special implications does the low fetal head have on the insertion process?

c.   What teaching will you provide regarding the preoperative and postoperative course?

78.   Janel's physician orders an IV. You insert an 18-gauge plastic cannula into the left forearm. The IV is to run at 150 cc/hr. The drop factor is 15 gtts/cc. You will set the drip rate at _____ gtts/min.

79.   Describe the location of the incision in the uterus and advantages and disadvantages of the following types of cesarean procedures.

a.   Low segment transverse

b.   Classic

80.   List the advantages and disadvantages of a low segment transverse and classic uterine incision.

a.   Low segment transverse

b.   Classic

81. As a part of Janel's preoperative nursing care, you identified Knowledge deficit related to lack of information about the postoperative course as an important nursing diagnosis. You establish the nursing goal "Provide information regarding the expected postoperative course" and select appropriate nursing interventions to accomplish this goal. Describe objective data that will show your teaching has been effective.

82. On her second postoperative day, Janel says to you, "I know that the cesarean was necessary and there was nothing that I did wrong but . . . why do I feel like I failed somehow?" What will you say?

Reflections

As you think about the clinical experiences you have had with childbearing women who were experiencing problems, what one woman or couple stands out in your mind? What were your feelings during that time? What type of problem was it? What was done to help? How did the situation turn out? How did the experience change you?

_____

_____

_____

_____

_____

_____

_____

_____

83.   Describe the teaching you might do to help a father feel more comfortable during a cesarean birth.

Vaginal Birth After Cesarean Birth (VBAC)

84.   Becky Saunders asks if she could have a vaginal birth next time even though she had a cesarean with her first birth.

   a.   Which contraindications should be assessed?

   b.   If she has a VBAC next time, she will be carefully assessed for which complications?

85.   **Critical Thinking Challenge:** The following situation has been included to challenge your critical thinking. Read the situation and then select one answer.

   Carla James, a 22-year-old gravida 2 para 1, had a cesarean birth last time. She has a vertical incision on her abdomen and asks, "Does this mean that I can have a VBAC next time?"

   Can Carla have a VBAC with her next birth?

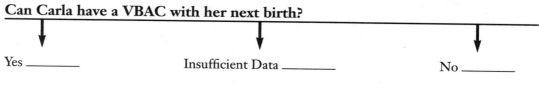

   Yes _____   Insufficient Data _____   No _____

   Explain your answer:

86.   **Memory Check:** Define the following abbreviations.

a.   AROM

b.   BPD

c.   CPD

d.   CS

e.   DIC

f.   ELF

g.   HELLP

h.   IUFD

i.   mec st

j.   Pit

k.   TOL

l.   VBAC

13 Newborn Physiologic Adaptation, Assessment, Needs and Care

This chapter corresponds to Chapters 21, 22, 23, and 24 in the 4th edition of *Maternal-Newborn Nursing Care: The Nurse, the Family, and the Community.*

Physiologic Adaptations

1. Describe four factors that are thought to stimulate the newborn to take its first breath.

   a.

   b.

   c.

   d.

2. State four anatomic and physiologic changes that occur in the cardiovascular system during the transition from fetal to neonatal circulation.

   a.

b.

c.

d.

3.   Newborn Zoe's temperature drops when she is placed on the cool plastic surface of the weight scales. This is an example of heat loss via

a.   conduction.

b.   convection.

c.   evaporation.

d.   radiation.

4.   What position do most newborns usually assume? Why?

5.   Describe the dialogue you would use to teach a new mother about physiologic jaundice. Include why the time of onset of the jaundice is important.

6. Discuss the expected level of development of the following senses in the newborn:

Sense	Assessment Method	Findings
Hearing		
Touch		
Taste/sucking		
Smell		
Pain		

Period of Reactivity

7. Which of the following behaviors are characteristic of the second period of reactivity?
   a. Awake and alert, lasts 4–6 hours, sucks, swallows
   b. Difficult to awaken, lasts 2–4 hours, bowel sounds present
   c. Eyes open, lasts 30 minutes, strong sucking reflex
   d. Face relaxed, regular and deep breaths, occasional startle

8. A primary nursing intervention appropriate to the second period of reactivity would be to
   a. auscultate the abdomen for the presence of bowel sounds.
   b. encourage the mother to begin breastfeeding.
   c. observe for excessive mucus.
   d. place infant under a radiant warmer.

ⓡeflections

Do you remember the first time you held and cared for a newborn in your mother-baby rotation? How did you feel? What were your thoughts/impressions?

_____

_____

_____

_____

_____

_____

_____

Gestational Age Assessment

As part of the admission process, the newborn's gestational age is determined. Using Ballard's gestational-age scoring tool (Figure 13–1 on page 161), determine Pam's gestational age.

Pam's gestational physical exam yields the following assessments of her physical maturity: her skin is cracking and has a pale area; some areas have no lanugo present; the breast bud is 1–2 mm with stippled areola; the ears are formed and firm with instant recoil; plantar creases extend over anterior two-thirds of sole; and the labia majora completely cover the minora and the clitoris. Assessment of Pam's neuromuscular development shows posture with flexion of the arms and hips, 0° square window, 90°–100° arm recoil, popliteal angle of 110°, scarf sign with elbow at midline, and a score of 4 for the head-to-ear maneuver.

Pam's birth weight was 3202 gm, her length was 49 cm, and her head circumference was 33.5 cm.

9.   Pam's Ballard score is (a) _____, which equates to a gestational age of

       (b) _____ weeks.

10.   Based on the gestational age you determined, correlate it with Pam's weight and classify her as

       LGA, AGA, or SGA. _____

       Plot Pam's length, weight, and head circumference on Figure 13–2 on page 162.

NEWBORN MATURITY RATING & CLASSIFICATION

ESTIMATION OF GESTATIONAL AGE BY MATURITY RATING
Symbols: X - 1st Exam   O - 2nd Exam

NEUROMUSCULAR MATURITY

	−1	0	1	2	3	4	5
Posture							
Square Window (wrist)	>90°	90°	60°	45°	30°	0°	
Arm Recoil		180°	140°–180°	110°–140°	90°–110°	<90°	
Popliteal Angle	180°	160°	140°	120°	100°	90°	<90°
Scarf Sign							
Heel to Ear							

PHYSICAL MATURITY

Skin	sticky friable transparent	gelatinous red, translucent	smooth pink, visible veins	superficial peeling &/or rash, few veins	cracking pale areas rare veins	parchment deep cracking no vessels	leathery cracked wrinkled
Lanugo	none	sparse	abundant	thinning	bald areas	mostly bald	
Plantar Surface	heel-toe 40–50mm:−1 <40mm:−2	>50mm no crease	faint red marks	anterior transverse crease only	creases ant. 2/3	creases over entire sole	
Breast	imperceptible	barely perceptible	flat areola no bud	stippled areola 1–2mm bud	raised areola 3–4mm bud	full areola 5–10mm bud	
Eye/Ear	lids fused loosely:−1 tightly:−2	lids open pinna flat stays folded	sl. curved pinna; soft; slow recoil	well curved pinna; soft but ready recoil	formed & firm instant recoil	thick cartilage ear stiff	
Genitals male	scrotum flat, smooth	scrotum empty faint rugae	testes in upper canal rare rugae	testes decending few rugae	testes down good rugae	testes pendulous deep rugae	
Genitals female	clitoris prominent labia flat	prominent clitoris small labia minora	prominent clitoris enlarging minora	majora & minora equally prominent	majora large minora small	majora cover clitoris & minora	

Scoring system: Ballard JL, Khoury JC, Wedig K, Wang L, Eilers-Walsman BL, Lipp R. New Ballard Score, expanded to include extremely premature infants *J Pediatr, 1991*; 119:417–423.

Gestation by Dates _____ wks

Birth Date _____ Hour _____ am/pm

APGAR _____ 1 min _____ 5 min

MATURITY RATING

score	weeks
−10	20
−5	22
0	24
5	26
10	28
15	30
20	32
25	34
30	36
35	38
40	40
45	42
50	44

SCORING SECTION

	1st Exam = X	2nd Exam = O
Estimating Gest Age by Maturity Rating	_____ Weeks	_____ Weeks
Time of Exam	Date _____ Hour _____ am/pm	Date _____ Hour _____ am/pm
Age at Exam	_____ Hours	_____ Hours
Signature of Examiner	_____ M.D.	_____ M.D.

Figure 13–1

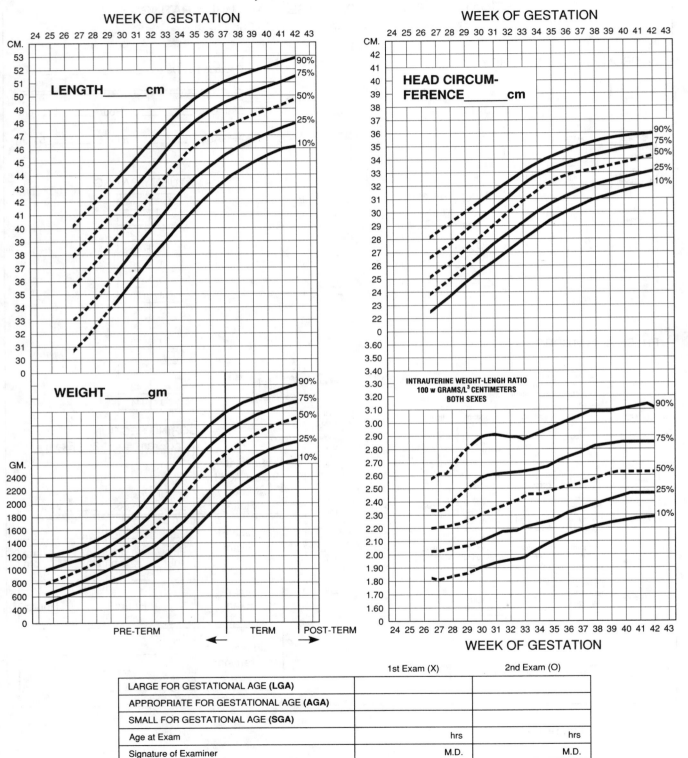

CLASSIFICATION OF NEWBORNS—
BASED ON MATURITY AND INTRAUTERINE GROWTH

Symbols: X-1st Exam O-2nd Exam

	1st Exam (X)	2nd Exam (O)
LARGE FOR GESTATIONAL AGE (LGA)		
APPROPRIATE FOR GESTATIONAL AGE (AGA)		
SMALL FOR GESTATIONAL AGE (SGA)		
Age at Exam	hrs	hrs
Signature of Examiner	M.D.	M.D.

Figure 13–2

11.   What factors might influence the neonate's gestational age score?

12.   Why is it important to determine the gestational age of all newborns?

Initial Assessments

13.   List the normal values for the following areas of initial assessment of the neonate:

Assessment Area	Normal Values
a. Temperature	
b. Pulse	
c. Respirations	
d. Blood pressure	
e. Average weight	
f. Average length	
g. Circumference of the head	
h. Circumference of the chest	

14.   Usual weight loss within the first 3–4 days of life for a full-term newborn is _____ percent.

15.   Why does the newborn commonly exhibit a "physiologic weight loss"?

16.   Draw dotted lines on Figure 13–3 to show where you would measure a newborn's head and chest.

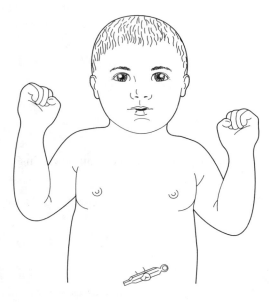

Figure 13–3   Measurement of newborn's head and chest.

17.   Describe how you would accurately and safely measure the newborn's length.

18.   Identify each of the following newborn skin variations, differentiating them by appearance, location, and significance:

a.   Harlequin color change

b.   Erythema neonatorum toxicum

c.   Telangiectatic nevi (stork bites)

d.   Nevus flammeus (port-wine stain)

e.   Mongolian spots

f.   Nevus vasculosus (strawberry mark)

19.   Which statement best defines a cephalhematoma?

   a.   Diffuse edema of the scalp resulting from compression of local blood vessels

   b.   Subperiosteal hemorrhage resulting from a traumatic birth

   c.   Temporary reshaping of the skull resulting from the pressure of birth

20.   On Figure 13–4, draw a series of numbered circles to indicate the correct sequence for auscultating a newborn's lungs. Place an "X" at the point where you should place your stethoscope in order to count the apical pulse.

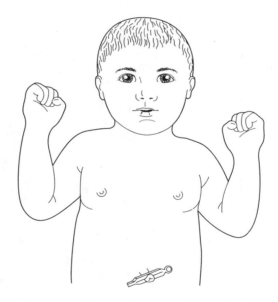

Figure 13–4   Auscultation of newborn's lungs and heart.

Physical Assessment of the Newborn

21.   As the newborn nurse, you would complete an initial physical assessment of each newborn. Complete the physical assessment chart on pp. 166–168.

Assessment Area	Normal Findings and Common Variations
Posture	
At rest	
Awake	
Skin	
Color	
Pigmentation	
Head	
Shape	
Sutures	
Fontanelles	
Face	
Eyes	
Movement	
Conjunctiva	
Ears	
Placement	
Nose	
Patency	

Assessment Area	Normal Findings and Common Variations
Mouth	
Gums	
Palate (hard & soft)	
Tongue	
Neck	
Clavicles	
Chest	
Shape	
PMI (point of maximal intensity)	
Characteristics of pulse	
Lungs	
Characteristics of breathing	
Cry	
Abdomen	
Umbilical cord vessels	
Hips	

→

Assessment Area	Normal Findings and Common Variations
Extremities Position	
Movement	
Genitalia	
Spine	
Anus Placement and patency	
Neuromuscular Movement and tone	

22.   The newborn is born with various reflexes. Complete the following chart:

Reflex	Description	How Elicited	Age at Disappearance
Moro			
Tonic neck			
Rooting			
Grasp			
Stepping			
Other			

23.   Identify four protective reflexes found in all normal newborns.

a.

b.

c.

d.

24.   As you complete the newborn physical assessment, alteration in findings may be identified. Describe the defining physical characteristics or alterations, and methods of assessment used for the following:

Hydrocephalus

Facial nerve palsy

Cleft palate

Omphalocele

Hypospadias

Myelomeningocele

Congenital dislocated hip

Clubfoot

25.   Why are the newborn's hands and feet often cold?

Care During Admission and First Four Hours of Life

You enter the birthing room to meet Ryan and his parents. Ryan is 20 minutes old and is in a quiet, alert state while interacting with his mother.

26.   What seven essential areas of information would you ascertain about Ryan's perinatal, intra-natal, and immediate postnatal period? Give your rationale.

a.

b.

c.

d.

e.

f.

g.

27.   List and prioritize eight nursing actions you would carry out during the first 4 hours (transitional period) of the newborn's life.

a.

b.

c.

d.

e.

f.

g.

h.

28.   Why is a vitamin K medication given prophylactically to newborns?

29.   **Critical Thinking in Practice:** The following action sequence is designed to help you think through basic clinical problems.

Glen, a 3450-gm baby boy, is born breech to Mrs Johns and has an Apgar score of 7 at 1 minute. Mrs Johns has requested to breastfeed Glen on the birthing bed.

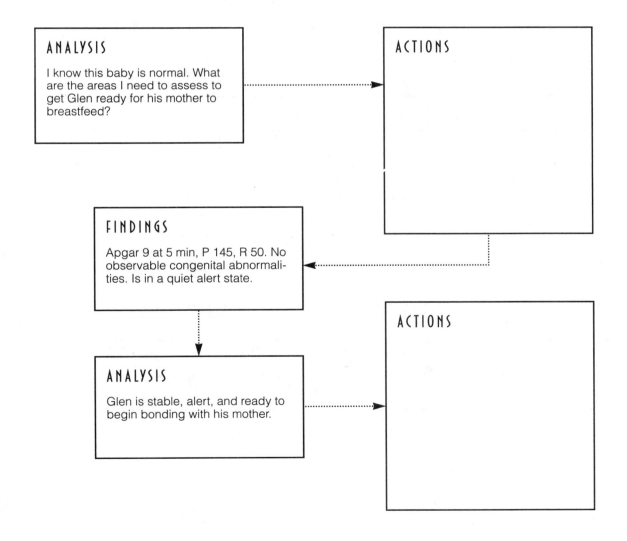

ANALYSIS

I know this baby is normal. What are the areas I need to assess to get Glen ready for his mother to breastfeed?

ACTIONS

FINDINGS

Apgar 9 at 5 min, P 145, R 50. No observable congenital abnormalities. Is in a quiet alert state.

ANALYSIS

Glen is stable, alert, and ready to begin bonding with his mother.

ACTIONS

30.   What is the appropriate dosage and preferred site for administration of vitamin K?

31.   Prophylactic eye ointments are instilled in the newborn's eyes in the immediate newborn period to prevent (a) _____, which is caused by (b) _____.

32.   List two prophylactic eye ointments that are commonly used.

      a.

      b.

33.   Write a sample newborn admission note.

_____

_____

_____

_____

_____

_____

_____

_____

_____

_____

_____

At the end of the transitional period, or 4–6 hours after birth, baseline laboratory tests are completed.

34.   For each of the following laboratory values, identify the significance and appropriate nursing interventions:

Laboratory Value	Significance	Nursing Interventions
Central hematocrit of 68%		
Hemoglobin of 12.5 gm/dL		
Bilirubin of 15 mg/dL		
Heelstick glucose <45 mg%		

35.   While working in the nursery, you notice that baby Ryan, age 5 hours, has turned blue. Closer inspection reveals a large amount of frothy mucus in his mouth. What would be your nursing diagnosis in this situation? What immediate nursing interventions would you undertake?

Ryan Montoya has successfully progressed through the transitional period; he is now 6 hours old and continues to be adapting well to extrauterine life.

Daily Newborn Nursing Assessments

36.   You are assigned to the mother-baby area. List seven daily assessments that are made of each newborn.

   a.

   b.

   c.

   d.

   e.

   f.

   g.

37.   Write a sample of a daily newborn nursing note.

_____

_____

_____

_____

_____

_____

_____

38.   Ryan is now 12 hours old. He voids as you begin to change his diaper. What observations should you make about his voiding?

39.   If Ryan had failed to void within 24 hours after birth, describe the assessments you would carry out.

40.   Within how many hours after birth would you expect Ryan to have his first stool and what would its appearance be?

Breastfeeding

41.   Helena Montoya wants to breastfeed Ryan. She tells you that she is really interested in breast-feeding but feels overwhelmed because she has so many questions and feels uncertain about beginning. She states, "I feel so full of questions that I wonder if I will ever know what to do." Based on your analysis of this data, formulate a nursing diagnosis that might apply.

42.   Based on your diagnosis, what information would you give Helena about breastfeeding her son?

   a.   Methods for encouraging the baby to nurse

   b.   Positions for feeding

   c.   Letdown reflex

   d.   Breaking suction before removing the infant from the breast

   e.   Length of time per breast

   f.   Frequency of feeding

43.   You stay and assist Helena with breastfeeding and answer her questions. Once she appears comfortable, you leave, but you check back with her periodically. Later in the morning when her baby is sleeping, you return to share information about other areas related to successful breastfeeding. What information would you share with Helena about the following areas?

a.   Nipple care

b.   Breast support

c.   Relief measures for breast engorgement

d.   Maternal nutrition while breastfeeding

e.   Environmental influences on successful breastfeeding

f.   Use of medications while breastfeeding

g.   Personal support systems

h.   Available community resources

44.   Helena is scheduled to remain on postpartum for only 24–48 hours. What actions can you take to help reinforce her learning so that things will go more smoothly when she is home?

45.   How will you evaluate the effectiveness of your teaching plan in meeting Helena's education needs?

46.   How would you evaluate the adequacy of Helena's fluid and nutritional intake while being breastfed?

Christy is a 2-day-old, bottle-fed, 3175-gm infant. During a follow-up call, her mother is concerned because "she takes only 1½ oz at each feeding."

47.   What would your response be?

48.   List at least five points to be included in a teaching plan to help Christy's mom successfully bottle-feed.

   a.

   b.

   c.

   d.

   e.

49.   On your mother-baby unit, you are conducting mothers' classes on newborn characteristics. The mothers express concerns about the following common occurrences. How would you respond to each?

   a.   "Can I hurt him by washing his hair over that soft spot? When will it close?"

   b.   "All my family's eyes are brown, but her eyes are blue."

c.   "Why are there tiny white spots across the bridge of her nose and on her chin?"

d.   "Are my baby's eyes all right? There are bright red marks on the white part of his eyes."

e.   "He has white patches in his mouth. Is that milk? How can you determine the cause?"

f.   "My son's breasts are so swollen. Will the swelling go down?"

g.   "When I changed her diaper, there was blood on it."

h.   "Are her feet clubbed? They turn in."

i.   "Why does his head look funny? The bones of his head cross over each other and look so narrow on the sides."

j.   List other questions you have been asked by mothers and your response to them.

Circumcision

50.   Prior to discharge, Ryan is circumcised. What are your nursing responsibilities during and following the circumcision?

51.   Nursing interventions for Ryan following his circumcision include

   a.   administering an analgesic.

   b.   applying a topical anesthetic to the site.

   c.   keeping him in the nursery for 1 hour.

   d.   loosely wrapping the diaper around him.

52.   Michael, an uncircumcised newborn, is ready for discharge. What instructions should you give his mother about penile care?

Discharge Teaching/Preparation for Care at Home

53.   You are to present a newborn discharge teaching program. List the essential components of this teaching program.

54.   Nursing actions that help a new mother identify her own baby after birth include

   a.   calling the infant by name as soon as possible after birth.

   b.   feeding the infant the first few times so that the mother can see the procedure.

   c.   strongly encouraging the mother to breastfeed.

   d.   undressing the baby completely so that all body parts can be seen.

55. Which of the following behaviors by a new father would indicate "engrossment"?

    a. Being able to express disappointment about the sex of the child

    b. Being afraid of hurting the infant while holding the infant

    c. Noting the individual characteristics of the infant including molding

    d. Stating that he feels more mature after seeing his infant for the first time

56. **Memory Check:** Define the following abbreviations.

    a. AC

    b. BAT

    c. CC

    d. HC

    e. PKU

14 Nursing Care of Newborns with Conditions Present at Birth

This chapter corresponds to Chapter 25 in the 4th edition of *Maternal-Newborn Nursing Care: The Nurse, the Family, and the Community.*

Classification of At-Risk Infants

1. Identify six maternal factors that may contribute to the birth of an at-risk infant.

    a.

    b.

    c.

    d.

    e.

    f.

Using a neonatal classification and mortality chart, plot each newborn's gestational age and weight, and identify the appropriate classification for each of the following newborns (each newborn may belong to a classification group based on both gestational age and weight):

2. Baby Joey is at 36–37 weeks' gestation, twin B, weighing 1500 gm.

    Classification _____

3. Baby Gwynn is at 42½ weeks' gestation by clinical determination and weighs 3150 gm.

    Classification _____

4.   Baby Sara is 34 weeks and weighs 2060 gm.

       Classification _____

5.   Baby Fernando is a 39-week newborn weighing 3950 gm.

       Classification _____

6.   Baby Carla is 41 weeks and weighs 2500 gm.

       Classification _____

7.   In assessing the newborn for at-risk status, the nurse should know that
       a.   any infant with a birth weight of less than 2500 grams is preterm.
       b.   the large-for-gestational-age infant has little risk of neonatal morbidity.
       c.   gestational age is the one criterion utilized to establish mortality risk.
       d.   infants who are preterm and small for gestational age have the highest mortality risk.

Small-for-Gestational-Age (SGA) Infant

8.   List four maternal causes for an SGA infant.

       a.

       b.

       c.

       d.

9.   What physical findings would you expect when scoring the gestational age of an SGA infant?

10.   Describe the potential complications associated with an SGA infant.

Infant of a Diabetic Mother (IDM)

11.   Richard is a 36 weeks' gestation newborn, weighing 9 lb 1 oz. His admitting nursery information indicates that his mother is a class C diabetic. What physical characteristics would you expect him to have?

12.   Identify the cause for Richard's large size.

13.   What laboratory test should be carried out on Richard and when?

14.   Richard may show beginning signs of hypoglycemia _____ hours after birth.

15.   Hypoglycemia occurs when blood glucose levels fall below _____ mg/dL.

16.   What signs of developing hypoglycemia would you observe in Richard? (See Chapter 26.)

17.   Identify the nursing interventions you would carry out relative to the assessment and treatment of hypoglycemia.

18.   Richard is a newborn who experienced symptomatic hypoglycemia and required an intravenous infusion of dextrose. His condition has stabilized and the physician has changed him to oral feedings. As Richard begins oral feedings, the nurse should anticipate that medical orders will include

    a.   discontinuing of IV after first formula feeding.

    b.   administering long-acting epinephrine.

    c.   giving a bolus infusion of 25% dextrose.

    d.   reinstituting frequent glucose monitoring during transition.

19. Infants of diabetic mothers are at risk for which of the following problems?

    a. Erythroblastosis fetalis

    b. Hypercalcemia

    c. Respiratory distress syndrome

    d. Seizures

20. Identify three other complications for which Richard is at risk.

Postterm Infant

21. List three obstetric indications of a postterm pregnancy.

    a.

    b.

    c.

22. Describe the clinical picture of a postterm infant.

23. Like the preterm infant, the newborn with postmaturity syndrome is at high risk for cold stress due to

    a. extended posture.

    b. absence of vernix.

    c. parchment-like skin.

    d. decreased subcutaneous fat.

24. Describe the potential complications for a postterm infant.

Preterm Infant

25.   List four major causes of prematurity.

a.

b.

c.

d.

26.   Which of the following characteristics is indicative of a preterm newborn of 34 weeks' gestation?

a.   The scalp hair is silky and lies in silky strands.

b.   The skin, except for the face, is covered with lanugo.

c.   The sole creases cover the anterior two-thirds of the foot.

d.   The upper two-thirds of the pinna curves inward.

27.   A preterm infant arrives in the nursery. What three initial assessments should you make?

a.

b.

c.

28.   When auscultating the chest of a preterm newborn the nurse hears rales and a continuous systolic murmur with clicks at the base of the heart. The nurse should suspect the presence of

a.   bronchopulmonary dysplasia.

b.   patent ductus arteriosus.

c.   pulmonary atelectasis.

d.   a ventricular septal defect.

29.   If an infant experiences an apneic episode, the first nursing activity should be to

a.   apply gentle tactile stimulation.

b.   call the physician.

c.   increase the rate of prescribed oxygen.

d.   suction the mouth and nose with a bulb syringe.

30.   The most common complication associated with preterm births is the development of

       a.   bronchopulmonary dysplasia.

       b.   periodic apnea.

       c.   persistent fetal circulation.

       d.   respiratory distress syndrome.

31.   Briefly describe the benefits of each: early breastmilk feedings (see Chapter 24) and premature
       formulas.

Mary, a 34-week preterm infant, is initially maintained on intravenous fluids via umbilical catheter.
When her respiratory status improves, she is placed on a half-strength premature formula via gavage
feedings every 2 hours.

32.   List three methods of assessing proper placement of a gavage tube prior to feedings.

       a.

       b.

       c.

33.   What nursing assessments would you make to determine the following?

       a.   Mary's tolerance of gavage feedings

       b.   Mary's readiness for nipple feeding

34. When Mary is two days old, her weight is average for gestational age (AGA). She is being carefully monitored prior to initiation of nipple feeding. Which of the following data groups would indicate that she is not ready for nipple feeding?

    a. Gaining weight; coordinated suck-swallow reflex

    b. Alert; axillary temperature of 97F

    c. Apical heart rate 120; skin temperature 36.5C

    d. Nasal flaring; sustained respiratory rate of 68

35. Briefly describe developmentally supportive nursing measures.

36. What would you do to facilitate attachment between parents and their at-risk infant?

37. What observations would you make in assessing the readiness of Mary's parents to take her home?

Infant of Substance-Abusing Mother

38. What common complications may be associated with cocaine-exposed infants?

39.   Claire, a 2-day-old, 3100-gm newborn, is observed to be going through withdrawal. Her 18-year-old mother was addicted to heroin during the pregnancy. List six symptoms of withdrawal you may observe in Claire.

a.

b.

c.

d.

e.

f.

40.   The nursing management of a heroin-addicted newborn experiencing withdrawal includes

a.   administration of methadone and frequent assessment of vital signs.

b.   frequent assessment of vital signs and wrapping the infant snugly in a blanket.

c.   meticulous skin and perineal care and frequent tactile stimulation.

d.   minimal tactile stimulation and the provision of loose, nonrestrictive clothing.

41.   During the past week, Claire has been irritable and eating poorly. She has not gained weight since birth. The physician orders phenobarbital for her. How many milligrams will the nurse administer per dose?

a.   6 mg

b.   12 mg

c.   24 mg

d.   36 mg

42.   What are the special needs of the drug-exposed infant at home?

Newborn at Risk for AIDS

43.   Nursing interventions for an infant at risk for AIDS include

    a.   a quiet, dim environment.

    b.   feeding with 24 cal/oz formula.

    c.   frequent, gentle handling.

    d.   tight swaddling.

44.   What instructions for care in the home should be given to parents of an infant at risk for AIDS?

Reflections

Think about an at-risk newborn you have taken care of. What were the parents' responses? Describe what the experience was like for you.

_____

_____

_____

_____

_____

_____

_____

45.   John is a newborn at risk for AIDS. John's parents are very anxious when they see him with all the special equipment around him. Your best response to facilitate parent-infant interaction would be to

a.   assure them that they are fortunate to have John in a special-care nursery.

b.   explain the equipment in simple terms, have them wash their hands, and provide an opportunity for them to touch John.

c.   explain the equipment simply and discuss the viability and continued existence of John.

d.   have them wash their hands so they can touch John.

46.   **Memory Check:** Define the following abbreviations.

a.   AIDS

b.   FAE

c.   FAS

d.   IDM

e.   ISAM

f.   IUGR

g.   LGA

h.   SGA

15 | Nursing Care of Newborns with Birth-Related Stressors

This chapter corresponds to Chapter 26 in the 4th edition of *Maternal-Newborn Nursing Care: The Nurse, the Family, and the Community.*

Resuscitation

Immediate newborn care for all at-risk newborns, in addition to providing warmth, is centered around determining the need for resuscitation.

1. Dava Walker has a previous obstetric history of fetal death of undetermined cause at 8 months' gestation. After the physician obtains a fetal scalp blood pH of 7.22, baby boy Walker is born. Which action by the nurse is the appropriate *initial* newborn resuscitation step?

   a. Inserting a nasogastric tube

   b. Suctioning the oro- and nasopharynx

   c. Inflating the lungs with positive pressure

   d. Positioning the head in the "sniffing position"

2. Baby Ken, a 43½-week postterm newborn, experienced early deceleration in labor. Yellow-green amniotic fluid was present at the time of membrane rupture.

   a. Ken is at risk for what neonatal problem?

   b. What resuscitative measures should be instituted as soon as his head and face appear on the perineum?

   c. What additional resuscitative measures or actions do you anticipate will be carried out after Ken is born?

3. **Critical Thinking Challenge:** The following situation has been included to challenge your critical thinking. Read the situation, then answer the question "yes" or "no," and give the rationale for your decision.

    Celeste, a 3200-gm term baby, is born vaginally. The amniotic fluid is lightly meconium stained. She was suctioned on the perineum and cried vigorously within 30 seconds of birth.

    Is Celeste a candidate for further resuscitation measures?

    Yes _____   No _____

    Explain your answer:

Brian, a term baby, was born vaginally 2 hours after his mother received 75 mg of Demerol IM. He has some flexion of extremities and acrocyanosis, HR-96, slow and irregular respiratory effort, and facial grimace. His Apgar at 1 min is 5. You are assisting the physician/neonatal nurse practitioner with the resuscitation.

4. Why is deep, vigorous suctioning of the airways to be avoided?

5. During bag-and-mask resuscitation you watch Brian's resuscitation bag to ensure it is inflating adequately, and you watch the pressure manometer to achieve the desired pressure of

    (a) _____ cm H_2O at a rate of (b) _____ times/min.

6. Based on Brian's intrapartal history, what other resuscitative measures does he need?

7. The first pharmacologic agent given in the chemical resuscitation phase of neonatal resuscitation is

   a. dopamine, to correct acidosis.

   b. epinephrine, to stimulate the heart.

   c. sodium bicarbonate, to correct acidosis.

   d. a volume expander, to maintain blood pressure.

On April 18 at 1:45 PM, a 35-week, 1580-gm male infant named Julio was born to a 20-year-old primigravida.

8. Julio is beginning to show signs of respiratory distress. Determine the priority for the following nursing interventions:

   1. Notify the physician.

   2. If cyanosis occurs, provide oxygen.

   3. Record time, symptoms, degree of symptoms, and whether oxygen relieved the symptoms of respiratory distress.

   4. Apply monitoring electrodes.

   5. Maintain a patent airway.

   a. 2, 1, 5, 4, and 3

   b. 5, 1, 2, 3, and 4

   c. 4, 2, 5, 1, and 3

   d. 5, 2, 1, 4, and 3

Respiratory Distress Syndrome

Tricia, a 3½ lb (1587 gm) newborn with a gestational age of 34 weeks, was born at 10:30 PM. Her Apgar score at 1 minute was 3, necessitating resuscitation via intubation and oxygen administration. On admission to the NICU, her vital signs are pulse 150, respirations 50, and rectal temperature of 96.2F (35.7C). She is placed in a radiant heat warmer, and an umbilical artery catheter is inserted for intravenous infusion.

9. You are to assess Tricia for signs of respiratory distress. List six signs indicative of developing respiratory distress.

   a.

   b.

   c.

   d.

   e.

   f.

10.   Additional physical assessment data on Tricia's respiratory status reveals minimal nasal flaring, chest lag on inspiration with just visible intercostal (lower chest) and xiphoid retractions, and audible expiratory grunting. Using the Silverman-Andersen index (Figure 15–1), your respiratory distress score for Tricia would be _____.

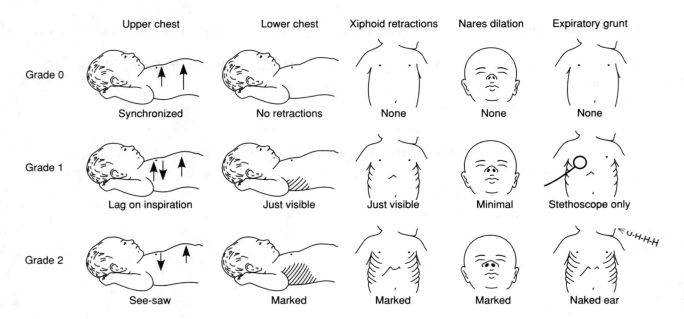

Figure 15–1 Evaluation of respiratory status using the Silverman-Andersen index. (From Ross Laboratories, Nursing Inservice Aid no. 2, Columbus, Ohio; and Silverman WA, Andersen DH: *Pediatrics* 1956:17:1. Copyright © 1956: American Academy of Pediatrics)

11.   What is the significance of Tricia's Silverman-Andersen score?

12.   What three factors may predispose Tricia to develop respiratory distress syndrome?

       a.

       b.

       c.

13.   It is now 2 AM, and Tricia is showing signs of respiratory distress syndrome. She is placed in an oxygen hood with a warmed, humidified oxygen concentration of 70 percent. What is the rationale for administering warmed and humidified oxygen?

14.   Tricia's respirations are now 65 per minute; she has an apical pulse of 152–176 beats per minute; and her arterial blood gases show a pH of 7.3, P_{O_2} of 55 mm Hg, and P_{CO_2} of 69 mm Hg. What are your nursing responsibilities during oxygen administration and how can you evaluate the effectiveness of the oxygen therapy?

15.   As Tricia's respiratory distress decreases, monitoring her respiratory status can be accomplished by noninvasive methods. Complete the following chart on noninvasive oxygen monitoring techniques.

Technique	Action	Nursing Responsibilities
Transcutaneous oxygen monitor (TCM)		
Pulse oximeter		

16.   Tricia's oxygen concentration is carefully regulated, based on her P_{O_2} and P_{CO_2} levels, because high blood levels of oxygen

  a.   cause cardiac shunt closures, although the latter are not permanent.

  b.   cause peripheral circulatory collapse.

  c.   may cause retinal spasms, leading to the development of retinopathy of prematurity.

  d.   may produce hyperbilirubinemia.

Cold Stress

At-risk infants are susceptible to temperature instability and should be placed in a regulated neutral thermal environment. If the infant's thermal environment is not maintained, cold stress can occur.

17.   What four metabolic changes and resultant problems may occur as a result of cold stress?

  a.

  b.

  c.

  d.

18.   Describe the nursing interventions you would institute to prevent or minimize hypothermia/cold stress.

19.   A small-for-gestational-age (SGA) newborn has experienced cold stress. Which of the following nursing actions should be included in the baby's care plan?

  a.   Using radiant warmer, institute measures for rapid temperature elevation

  b.   Initiate dextrostix monitoring of blood glucose levels

  c.   Monitor rectal temperature hourly

  d.   Rapidly infuse 50% dextrose IV per standing protocol (or obtain order for)

Neonatal Jaundice

20.   List three factors that influence the rate and amount of bilirubin conjugation.

a.

b.

c.

21.   State three situations that alter the newborn's ability to conjugate bilirubin.

a.

b.

c.

22.   Identify the characteristics of pathologic jaundice as related to causes, time of onset, and bilirubin level in the term and preterm newborn.

23.   What factors might influence your assessment of the newborn's developing jaundice?

24.   An African-American mother asks how to assess for jaundice in her newborn. Which of the following is the most appropriate answer for the nurse to offer?

   a.   "A good place to look is the inside of the mouth. Use a good light to help you see."

   b.   "Pressing the sole of your baby's foot is helpful. If it blanches yellow, then the baby is considered jaundiced."

   c.   "The best way to assess your baby is to check the white part of the eyes. If jaundice is present, they will have a yellow color."

   d.   "Such an assessment is best done by the doctor. She knows how to identify jaundice."

25. **Critical Thinking in Practice:** The following action sequence is designed to help you think through a clinical problem pertaining to hemolytic disease of the newborn.

You are taking care of Alice, a 24-hour-old, 7 lb 2 oz newborn, and her mother on the mother-baby unit. During your initial assessments and care of Alice, you notice she looks yellow.

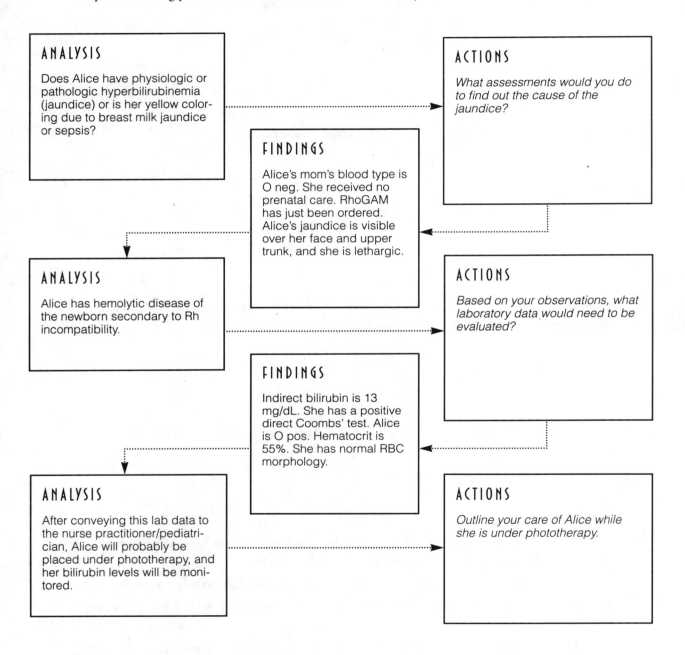

ANALYSIS

Does Alice have physiologic or pathologic hyperbilirubinemia (jaundice) or is her yellow coloring due to breast milk jaundice or sepsis?

ACTIONS

What assessments would you do to find out the cause of the jaundice?

FINDINGS

Alice's mom's blood type is O neg. She received no prenatal care. RhoGAM has just been ordered. Alice's jaundice is visible over her face and upper trunk, and she is lethargic.

ANALYSIS

Alice has hemolytic disease of the newborn secondary to Rh incompatibility.

ACTIONS

Based on your observations, what laboratory data would need to be evaluated?

FINDINGS

Indirect bilirubin is 13 mg/dL. She has a positive direct Coombs' test. Alice is O pos. Hematocrit is 55%. She has normal RBC morphology.

ANALYSIS

After conveying this lab data to the nurse practitioner/pediatrician, Alice will probably be placed under phototherapy, and her bilirubin levels will be monitored.

ACTIONS

Outline your care of Alice while she is under phototherapy.

26. A newborn undergoing phototherapy experiences increased urine output and loose stools. The nurse should

    a. institute enteric isolation.

    b. immediately discontinue phototherapy.

    c. decrease the phototherapy unit's level of irradiance.

    d. observe for clinical manifestations of dehydration.

27. While receiving phototherapy babies should

    a. be unclothed with the eyes shielded.

    b. be unclothed with the eyes and genitals shielded.

    c. not be removed from under the lights until treatment is completed.

    d. not be disturbed by frequent parental visits.

Newborn with Polycythemia

28. For a newborn with polycythemia, which of the following laboratory results would indicate that medical therapy is effective?

    a. Central venous hematocrit of 70%

    b. Central venous hematocrit of 55%

    c. Venous hemoglobin of 25 g/dL

    d. Serum calcium level of 8.0 mg/dL

Neonatal Infections

29. You are taking care of Haruko, who is 2 days old, and you note that he is increasingly lethargic and refuses to eat. He is diagnosed as having sepsis neonatorum. List four factors that increase the newborn's susceptibility to infections.

    a.

    b.

    c.

    d.

30. Identify three bacterial organisms that may cause sepsis neonatorum.

a.

b.

c.

31. In newborns, an early sign of sepsis is
a. hypothermia.
b. hyperglycemia.
c. jitteriness.
d. tachycardia.

32. Identify four diagnostic tests that might be done in a septic workup.

a.

b.

c.

d.

33. What are your nursing responsibilities while caring for a septic newborn? Include your rationale.

34. The most common congenitally acquired viral infection is
a. cytomegalovirus.
b. herpes simplex virus.
c. syphilis.

35.   **Memory Check:** Define the following abbreviations.

    a.   BPD

    b.   MAS

    c.   RDS

    d.   TNZ

    e.   UAC

16 | Nursing Assessment and Care of the Postpartal Family

This chapter corresponds to Chapters 27 and 28 in the 4th edition of *Maternal-Newborn Nursing Care: The Nurse, the Family, and the Community*.

1. Define *postpartum*.

Attachment Immediately After Birth

2. Lisa and George just had their first baby 10 minutes ago. What stage of labor and birth are they in?

3. Lisa and George are exhibiting beginning attachment behaviors. What will you observe?

4. How can you support the attachment process at this time?

Physiologic Postpartal Changes

5.   The fundus should be

    a.   at the level of the symphysis pubis.

    b.   at the level of the umbilicus.

    c.   midway between the umbilicus and symphysis pubis.

    d.   two fingerbreadths below the umbilicus.

6.   The lochia should have a

    a.   characteristic foul odor and be blood mixed with a small amount of mucus.

    b.   characteristic foul odor and be dark brown with occasional red bleeding.

    c.   fleshy odor and be clear-colored and moderate in amount.

    d.   fleshy odor with blood and a small amount of mucus mixed in.

7.   The perineum should be

    a.   edematous, painful to pressure, and displaying a clear discharge.

    b.   edematous, painful to pressure, and perhaps displaying hemorrhoids.

    c.   intensely painful in the episiotomy area and displaying clear drainage.

    d.   displaying clear drainage and perhaps hemorrhoids.

8.   The breasts should be

    a.   filling and secreting colostrum.

    b.   engorged and secreting colostrum.

    c.   soft and secreting milk.

    d.   engorged and not secreting any fluid.

9.   Uterine involution occurs as a result of

    a.   a decrease in the number of myometrial cells.

    b.   necrosis of the hypertrophic myometrial cells.

    c.   autolysis of protein material within the uterine wall.

    d.   necrotic degeneration of the placental site.

10.   Explain the physiologic mechanisms that cause each of the following:

    a.   Postpartal chill

→

b.   Postpartal diaphoresis

c.   Afterpains

11.   During the postpartal period, what psychologic adaptations does a new mother face?

12.   Describe "postpartum blues."

Maternal Role Attainment

13.   Name and briefly describe the four stages of maternal role attainment.

a.

b.

c.

d.

Assessment of the Postpartal Woman

14. Identify nine areas that should be examined during the initial postpartal *physical* assessment and then at least daily until the woman is discharged. (Do not include psychologic assessment or information needs.)

    a.

    b.

    c.

    d.

    e.

    f.

    g.

    h.

    i.

15. Describe three observations you should make in assessing the breasts of a woman postpartally. Include your rationale for each.

    a.

    b.

    c.

16.   The fundus is assessed following childbirth.

   a.   Why is it necessary?

   b.   Why is the client asked to empty her bladder before you assess her fundus?

   c.   Describe the correct procedure for evaluating descent of the fundus.

   d.   How is fundal height recorded (according to your agency's policy)?

17.   Soon Yee, a 21-year-old primipara, gave birth 4 hours ago. Immediately following birth her fundus was midway between the symphysis and the umbilicus. Where would you expect it to be now?

18.   What characteristics should you note in assessing Soon's lochia?

19.   How do you record your findings about her lochia (according to your agency's policy)?

20.   Soon reports that she got up to the bathroom a short time ago and noticed a sudden increase in her lochia. From your check you know that her fundus is firm. How would you explain this occurrence to her?

21.   In preparation for assessing Soon's perineum, you would have her assume the

        _____ position.

22.   What observations about the condition of the client's anal area should be made during the assessment of the perineum?

23.   What information regarding the client's urinary elimination should you elicit during your physical assessment?

24.   What information about your client's intestinal elimination should you elicit during your physical assessment?

25.   Discuss the teaching implications of your findings on intestinal elimination.

26.   Why is it important to include an evaluation of your client's lower extremities as part of your postpartal assessment?

27.   How is Homan's sign elicited?

28.	**Critical Thinking in Practice:** The following action sequence is designed to help you think through basic clinical problems.

Margo Jessup gave birth at 0400. At 0830 you are completing her morning postpartum assessment. You find her fundus at one fingerbreadth above the umbilicus and displaced to the right side.

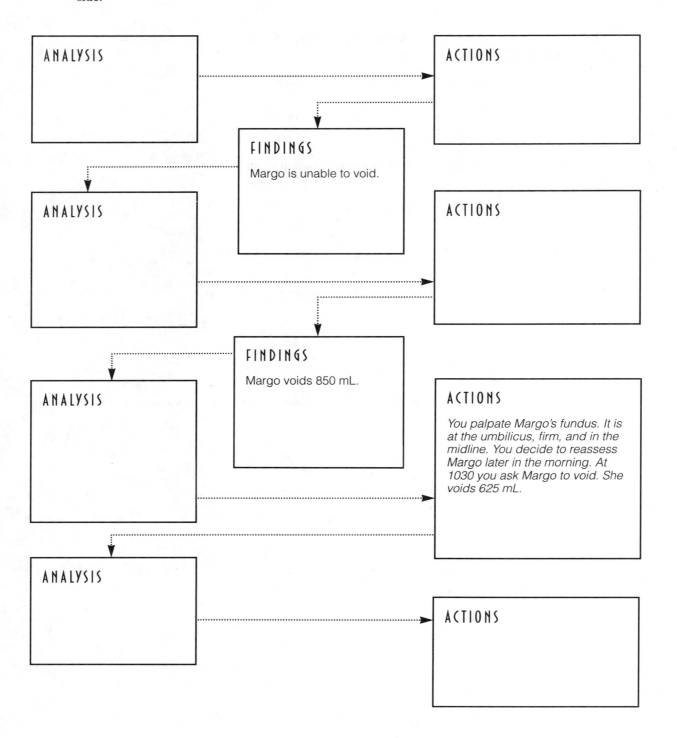

ANALYSIS

ACTIONS

FINDINGS

Margo is unable to void.

ANALYSIS

ACTIONS

FINDINGS

Margo voids 850 mL.

ANALYSIS

ACTIONS

You palpate Margo's fundus. It is at the umbilicus, firm, and in the midline. You decide to reassess Margo later in the morning. At 1030 you ask Margo to void. She voids 625 mL.

ANALYSIS

ACTIONS

Reflections

Think about a woman you have cared for postpartally or someone you have visited soon after the birth of a child (perhaps this may apply to you). What were her emotions like? Did she share her feelings with you? Did she show any signs of the postpartum blues?

_____

_____

_____

_____

_____

_____

_____

_____

_____

29.   What assessments are important in evaluating your client's nutritional status?

30.   Discuss factors you should consider in completing a psychologic assessment postpartally.

Relief of Postpartal Discomforts

31.   For each of the discomforts listed below, identify two comfort measures.

    a.   Episiotomy

    b.   Hemorrhoids

    c.   Afterpains

Suppression of Lactation

32.   Suppression of lactation in nonnursing mothers is generally accomplished by mechanical methods. Explain these methods.

33.   You are assisting Edna Lewis to the bathroom for the first time following childbirth.

    a.   What nursing assessments should you make before Edna gets up?

    b.   What teaching regarding perineal hygiene should you initiate at this time?

    c.   Edna decides to remain in the bathroom and take a shower after she voids. What precautions should you take to ensure her safety?

34.   During the postpartal period, you may be asked to administer rubella. Describe the action/use, dose, side effects/untoward effects, and nursing considerations.

Psychologic Responses

35.   Identify factors that influence a new mother's psychologic adjustment to childbirth and her newborn.

36.   How can a nurse provide emotional support during this time?

37.   You are caring for a woman who gave birth to a healthy infant 5 hours ago. When you enter her room, she is crying. She states, "I don't know what's wrong with me. I feel as let down as if it were the day after Christmas, and I can't seem to stop crying. What's going on? Do you know why I'm acting like this?" How would you respond?

38.   Freda and Earl Marshall express concern about the possible reaction of their 3-year-old son Roy to the birth of their daughter. Briefly describe some actions they might take to help Roy more easily adjust to the arrival of his sister.

39. In many postpartal units the focus of care and attention is the mother and her newborn. Describe how you would incorporate the father or support person into your focus of care.

40. In addition to her name, age, and social history, what information would you consider essential to have as part of your database in planning care for a woman postpartally?

41. Carla Roberts, age 29, gravida 3 para 2, gave birth to an 8 lb 7 oz boy at 4:15 AM. Her labor lasted 18 hours, and the baby was born by low forceps. She received no medication during labor but did have a pudendal block for birth. She had a midline episiotomy and a third-degree extension. She also has two large hemorrhoids. The baby had an Apgar score of 7 at 1 minute and 9 at 5 minutes. He is apparently healthy, although he has a large bruise on each temple from the forceps and pronounced molding of his head. The labor nurse reported that Harry Roberts, Carla's husband, was present at the birth and expressed great pleasure at the birth of his third son. Carla was openly disappointed that the newborn was not the girl she had so greatly desired.

It is now 8 AM. Carla has just finished breakfast, and you are assigned as her nurse today. Carla has voided twice since birth: 700 mL and 550 mL. Her fundus has remained firm and is at the umbilicus. Her lochia is rubra and moderate. Her vital signs are normal, and she is a breast-feeding mother. Her orders include a shower; a sitz bath tid; Dermaplast spray prn; up ad lib; Tylenol #3 q4h prn; a regular diet; fluids; a straight catheter × 1 prn for marked distention; and Surfak 1 capsule bid. She is to be discharged at noon unless complications arise.

a. What do you consider the highest priorities in planning Carla's physical care?

b. What behaviors might Carla exhibit that would suggest possible failure to attach?

Postpartal Care of the Woman Following Cesarean Birth

42.   How does postpartum assessment and care differ for the woman who gives birth by cesarean?

43.   Patient-controlled analgesia (PCA) is becoming increasingly popular.

   a.   Describe how it is used.

   b.   How is the client on PCA protected from overdose?

Care of the Adolescent Mother

44.   Describe some of the special nursing needs of the adolescent mother postpartally.

45.   How can the postpartum nurse provide support and assistance to a woman who is relinquishing her infant?

Discharge Teaching

46.   Vicky and Larry Darnell are preparing to take their first child, Lori, home at 2:00 PM. Vicky is planning to bottle-feed Lori. Vicky had an uncomplicated labor and birth but has a small midline episiotomy that has caused some discomfort. You are assigned to Mrs Darnell today and are responsible for discharge teaching. Describe what information you will include in your discharge teaching for the following areas:

a.   Care of the episiotomy

b.   Rest

c.   Activity and exercises

d.   Resumption of sexual activity and birth control methods

e.   Symptoms in the mother that should be reported

f.   Support systems

g. Baby care

h. Symptoms in the baby that should be reported

i. Infant safety (crib, car seat)

j. Follow-up medical care for both mother and infant

k. Community resources

47. LaTisha Carson gave birth to her first child in the birthing room 6 hours ago. Now she is preparing for discharge. Describe how you will explain the reasons for and importance of returning to the hospital for a test for phenylketonuria and other metabolic disorders.

17 | Home Care of the Postpartal Family

This chapter corresponds to Chapter 29 in the 4th edition of *Maternal-Newborn Nursing Care: The Nurse, the Family, and the Community.*

Home Visits

1. The three areas of focus for a home visit to a postpartal family include

    a.

    b.

    c.

2. How is a postpartal home visit different from community health visits?

3. Identify five actions a nurse should take to ensure personal safety during a home visit.

    a.

    b.

    c.

    d.

    e.

4. What should the nurse do if he or she begins to feel unsafe during a home visit?

Home Care of the Newborn

5. Which of the following holding methods is recommended when shampooing the infant?

    a. cradle hold

    b. football hold

    c. upright position

6. Why should the infant's resting position be changed periodically, especially during the early months of life?

7. Identify at least two reasons for positioning a newborn infant on her or his side.

    a.

    b.

8. You are on a home visit to Elena Espinoza and her newborn daughter, Rose. Mrs Espinoza asks when she can switch from sponge baths to tub baths. How would you respond?

9. What information should you give Mrs Espinoza about assessment and care of Rose's umbilical cord?

10.   The newborn's temperature should be taken by the _____ route.

For each of the following statements about newborn care, indicate **T** if the statement is true and **F** if it is false.

11.   _____   Newborns should be given a daily bath.

12.   _____   The eyes are washed from the inner to the outer canthus.

13.   _____   The ear canal should be cleaned regularly with a cotton swab.

14.   _____   Talcum powder is applied generously to help keep the infant's skin dry.

15.   _____   The genital area should be cleansed daily with soap and water and with water after each wet or dirty diaper.

16.   _____   The foreskin of uncircumcised infants should be gently retracted each day.

17.   _____   If necessary, the newborn's nails may be trimmed straight across.

18.   Complete the following chart comparing the stools of breastfed and formula-fed infants:

Characteristics of Stools	Breastfed	Formula-Fed
Frequency		
Color		
Consistency		
Odor		

Home Care of the Postpartal Woman and Family

19.   List four physical and developmental tasks the new mother must accomplish during the postpartal period.

    a.

    b.

    c.

    d.

20.   Summarize areas of assessment the nurse should complete on the new mother during a pospartal home visit.

    a.   Physical assessment

    b.   Psychosocial assessment

For each of the following physical findings in the postpartal woman, indicate with a "**1**" those that are normally found at the first postpartal home visit and with a "**6**" those that are normally found by six weeks postpartum.

21.   _____   Weight loss of 30 lb

22.   _____   Abdominal musculature somewhat lax

23.   _____   Striae pink and readily apparent

24.   _____   Nonnursing mother: breasts firm to the touch

25.   _____   Normal bowel elimination pattern

26.   _____   Lochia serosa, scant

27.   _____   Fundus not palpable above symphysis

28.   During a home visit, you assess a new mother for signs of bonding with her infant. List at least five signs that might indicate a failure to bond.

      a.

      b.

      c.

      d.

      e.

18 | The Postpartal Family at Risk

This chapter corresponds to Chapter 30 in the 4th edition of *Maternal-Newborn Nursing Care: The Nurse, the Family, and the Community.*

Postpartum Hemorrhage

1. Postpartum hemorrhage may be classified as early or late. Describe the time of onset and primary cause(s) of each.

    a. Early

    b. Late

Joan Taranta, a 33-year-old gravida 3 para 3, is recovering following the birth of twin boys. Her labor lasted 2½ hours.

2. Identify two factors that predispose Joan to early postpartum hemorrhage.

    a.

    b.

3. During your assessment of Joan, what three findings would indicate possible postpartum hemorrhage?

    a.

    b.

    c.

4. Your nursing assessment indicates that Joan is having an early postpartum hemorrhage. Formulate an appropriate nursing diagnosis.

5. What do you consider the two highest priorities in planning your care of Joan?

6. The nurse finds Joan's uterus to be boggy, high, and deviated to the right. The most appropriate nursing action is to

   a. have Joan void and then re-evaluate the fundus.

   b. massage the uterus and re-evaluate in 30 minutes.

   c. notify the physician.

   d. place Joan on a pad count.

7. What additional nursing interventions should be initiated for Joan as she demonstrates signs of postpartum hemorrhage?

8. A client who has an estimated blood loss of 1300 mL 8 hours postbirth is said to have

   a. mild, early postpartum hemorrhage.

   b. severe, early postpartum hemorrhage.

   c. mild, late postpartum hemorrhage.

   d. severe, late postpartum hemorrhage.

9.   **Critical Thinking in Practice:** The following action sequence is designed to help you think through basic clinical problems.

You are taking care of Mrs Carrie Spencer, age 24, G1 P1, on the mother-baby unit. She is 8 hours postbirth of an 8 lb 2 oz baby girl. As you are carrying out her postpartal assessments, she complains of tenderness and pain in her perineal area. She says, "My stitches hurt; it feels as if they are tearing apart."

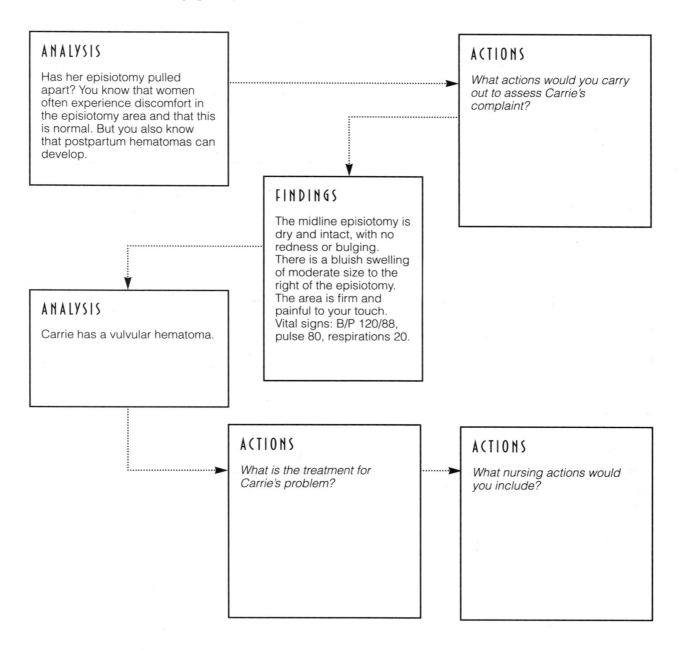

ANALYSIS

Has her episiotomy pulled apart? You know that women often experience discomfort in the episiotomy area and that this is normal. But you also know that postpartum hematomas can develop.

ACTIONS

What actions would you carry out to assess Carrie's complaint?

FINDINGS

The midline episiotomy is dry and intact, with no redness or bulging. There is a bluish swelling of moderate size to the right of the episiotomy. The area is firm and painful to your touch. Vital signs: B/P 120/88, pulse 80, respirations 20.

ANALYSIS

Carrie has a vulvular hematoma.

ACTIONS

What is the treatment for Carrie's problem?

ACTIONS

What nursing actions would you include?

Reflections

Have you provided care for a woman experiencing bleeding in the immediate postpartum period? What concerns did she express? Describe the experience.

_____

_____

_____

_____

_____

_____

_____

_____

_____

_____

Subinvolution

Mrs Gloria Brown, a breastfeeding mother, gave birth to a 8 lb 11½ oz baby boy, Vincent, vaginally after Pitocin augmentation. She has been home for 2 weeks and calls the office. She tells the Ob/Gyn nurse practitioner that she is concerned because her flow has increased and is red but not foul smelling.

10.   Identify nursing assessments that might lead you to suspect subinvolution.

11.   Identify three nursing interventions to meet Mrs Brown's needs.

Postpartal Reproductive Tract Infections

12.   The clinical manifestations of a localized infection of the episiotomy would include

   a.   approximation of skin edges of the episiotomy.

   b.   client complaint of severe discomfort in the perineum and an oral temperature of 99.8F (37.7C).

   c.   reddened, bruised tissue.

   d.   reddened, edematous tissue with yellowish discharge.

Rich and Kim James have delivered their third baby by cesarean birth.

13.   The nurse's assessment of Kim reveals an elevation in her temperature, chills, nausea, and increased pain. The nurse notifies the primary physician and receives the following orders: ampicillin in 500 mg IV q6h, culture and sensitivity of lochia, ultrasound of the pelvis, and chest x-ray. Which order should the nurse carry out first?

   a.   Ultrasound

   b.   IV antibiotic

   c.   Culture of lochia

   d.   Chest x-ray

14.   Kim's incision has become infected and she has been placed in isolation. Since the baby can no longer room-in, how can the nurse promote bonding between Kim and her infant?

   a.   Provide a picture of the baby for Kim.

   b.   Have Rich visit the baby more often.

   c.   Assure Kim she will be in isolation only a short time.

   d.   Encourage Kim to use the time away from the baby to rest so she will recover faster.

15.   Complete the following chart on puerperal infection:

Component	Localized Infection (Episiotomy and/or Laceration)	Endometritis (Metritis)	Pelvic Cellulitis (Parametritis)
Tissues involved			
Clinical manifestations			
Interventions			
Complications			

16.   Identify evaluative outcome criteria findings that indicate your interventions/treatments of puerperal infection have been effective.

17.   What home care instructions would you give a mother about puerperal infections?

Thromboembolic Diseases

18.   Discuss the physiologic changes of pregnancy that increase a woman's susceptibility to blood clot formation during the postpartal period.

Match the following descriptive statements with the correct thromboembolic disease.

19. _____ Clotting process involving the saphenous vein system

    a.   Superficial thrombophlebitis

20. _____ More frequently seen in women with history of thrombosis

    b.   Deep vein thrombosis (DVT)

21. _____ Usually appears about third or fourth postpartal day

    c.   Pulmonary embolism

22. _____ Sudden onset of sweating, pallor, dyspnea, and chest pain

23. _____ Prompt intervention with heparin, oxygen, and lidocaine as needed

24. _____ Edema of ankle and leg; low-grade fever and positive Homan's sign

25. _____ Treatment primarily involves intravenous heparin and bed rest

26. _____ Management principally involves leg elevation, moist packs, bed rest, and elastic stockings

27. Identify three interventions useful in preventing the development of thrombophlebitis during the postpartal period.

a.

b.

c.

28. Describe the appropriate interventions for a mother with deep vein thrombosis.

Marie LaCoste has recently given birth and states that she has a history of thrombophlebitis.

29. Which of the following nursing measures will be most important for Marie in light of her history?

   a. Assess vital signs frequently.

   b. Encourage early ambulation.

   c. Encourage Marie to rest in bed with the knee gatch up.

   d. Maintain bed rest.

30. Marie has developed thrombophlebitis and is receiving heparin intravenously. It will be important to watch her for signs of overdose, which include

   a. dysuria.

   b. epistaxis, hematuria, and dysuria.

   c. hematuria, ecchymosis, and epistaxis.

   d. hematuria, ecchymosis, and vertigo.

31. The antagonist of heparin is _____.

32. A positive Homan's sign is indicated by a complaint of pain in

   a. the foot when the client stands.

   b. the leg when the foot is dorsiflexed while the knee is held flat.

   c. the leg when the knee is flexed and the foot is extended.

   d. the leg when the knee is held flat and the foot is rotated.

33. What education for self-care at home should be given to a woman receiving warfarin (Coumadin)?

34.   **Critical Thinking Challenge:** The following situation has been included to challenge your critical thinking. Read the situation, answer the question "yes" or "no," and give your rationale.

Jeanne McGuire, age 34, G3 P3, gave birth to twin boys vaginally with regional anesthesia 12 hours ago and you are now responsible for her care. She complains of cramping when the uterus attempts to contract. Your assessment reveals a uterus one fingerbreadth above the umbilicus and displaced to the right, and increased vaginal bleeding.

Is Mrs McGuire a candidate for bladder distention?

Yes _____   No _____

Explain your answer:

Puerperal Cystitis

35.   List three factors that predispose the postpartal woman to the development of cystitis.

a.

b.

c.

36.   Identify appropriate interventions in the treatment of the postpartal woman with cystitis.

Mastitis

One week after her discharge, Alice Enriquez, a 23-year-old gravida 1 para 1 breastfeeding mother, develops mastitis.

37.   List two factors that contribute to the development of mastitis.

   a.

   b.

38.   Identify four clinical manifestations of mastitis that Alice may exhibit.

   a.

   b.

   c.

   d.

Two nursing diagnoses that may apply to Alice are Acute pain related to inflammation and swelling of breast tissue and Knowledge deficit related to lack of information about appropriate breastfeeding techniques.

39.   Based on these possible nursing diagnoses, describe the interventions that Alice or you may institute.

40.   In evaluating the nursing diagnosis Knowledge deficit related to lack of information about appropriate breastfeeding techniques, identify the evaluative outcome criteria that would indicate that Alice's knowledge about breastfeeding during mastitis has changed.

Postpartal Mood Disorders

It is the third postpartal day for Bonnie Sumpter, an 18-year-old primipara. She is single and is keeping her baby. The nurse makes a home visit and expresses concern that Bonnie may not be bonding appropriately with her infant.

41.   Identify four feelings or behaviors that might indicate "postpartum blues."

      a.

      b.

      c.

      d.

Epilogue

By now you are probably almost finished with your maternity rotation. We hope this workbook has helped you focus your study so that you are more comfortable in relating your knowledge of theory to your clinical practice. We believe that in this way you will be better nurses, and that the childbearing families for whom you are responsible will receive better care.

1 | Answer Key

1. (a) The RNC has shown expertise in a field by taking a national certification examination; (b) The CNS has a master's degree and specialized knowledge and competence in a specific clinical area; (c) The NP has received specialized education in a master's degree program or certificate program and can function in an advanced practice role; (d) The CNM is educated as both a nurse and a midwife and is certified by the American College of Nurse-Midwives.
2. b
3. See text, p. 8
4. (a) Number of live births per 1000 people; (b) number of deaths of infants under 1 year of age per 1000 live births in a given population; (c) number of deaths of infants less than 28 days of age per 1000 live births; (d) number of deaths from any cause during the pregnancy cycle (including the 42-day postpartal period) per 100,000 live births.
5. Answers include: increased use of hospitals and specialized health care personnel by maternity clients; improved high-risk care for mothers and infants; prevention and control of infection with antibiotics and improved techniques; availability of blood and blood products for transfusions; lowered rates of anesthesia-related deaths.
6. d
7. See text, p. 9

2 | Answer Key

1. a
2. c
3. b
4. e
5. f
6. d
7. See text, p. 19, Figure 2–2
8. The vagina serves as a passageway for sperm, fetal delivery, and the products of menstruation. It protects against trauma from sexual intercourse and infection.
9. Factors that can destroy the self-cleansing ability of the vagina include antibiotic therapy, douching, and use of perineal sprays or deodorants.
10. (a) isthmus of fallopian tube, (b) uterine cavity, (c) uterine body, (d) endometrium, (e) myometrium, (f) internal os, (g) isthmus, (h) cervix, (i) vagina
11. b
12. The endometrium produces a thin, watery, alkaline secretion that helps sperm travel to the fallopian tubes; it nourishes the developing embryo prior to implantation.
13. (a) lubricates vaginal canal, (b) acts as a bacteriostatic action, (c) provides an alkaline environment to protect sperm from the acidic vagina
14. b
15. See text, pp. 22–23
16. The fallopian tubes provide: transport for the ovum from the ovary to the uterus (which takes 3–4 days); a site for fertilization; and a warm, moist, nourishing environment for the ovum and zygote.
17. See text, pp. 23–24
18. See text, p. 24
19. The ovaries secrete estrogen and progesterone and are responsible for ovulation.
20. See text, p. 25, Figure 2–8
21. See text, p. 26, Figure 2–9
22. levator ani

23. (a) Portion above pelvic brim or linea terminalis; supports the pregnant uterus; directs the presenting fetal part into true pelvis below. (b) Lies below linea terminalis; its shape and size determines adequacy of birth passage. (c) Upper border of true pelvis; usually rounded; determines whether engagement can occur. (d) Lower border of the true pelvis; if too narrow the baby's head may be pushed backward, making extension difficult and causing shoulder dystocia for large babies.
24. (a) false pelvis, (b) true pelvis, (c) pelvic inlet, (d) pelvic outlet
25. See text, p. 29, Figure 2–13
26. The tubercles of Montgomery secrete a fatty substance that helps lubricate and protect the breasts.
27. a
28. (a) ovarian, (b) menstrual
29. See text, pp. 29–32
30. c
31. a
32. *Follicular phase:* under the influence of FSH, the graafian follicle matures; LH assists the oocyte in rupturing out of the ovary around day 14. *Luteal phase:* after rupture, the corpus luteum (CL) forms; if fertilization does not occur, the CL degenerates and progesterone and estrogen decreases, which results in menses.
33. See text, pp. 33–34
34. See text, p. 30, Figure 2–14
35. a
36. (a) penis, (b) epididymides, (c) vas deferens, (d) testes, (e) testis, (f) Leydig's cells, (g) seminiferous tubules, (h) Sertoli's, (i) seminal vesicles, (j) ejaculatory duct, (k) prostate, (l) seminal fluid, (m) bulbourethral (Cowper's)
37. (a) female reproductive cycle, (b) follicle-stimulating hormone, (c) gonadotropin-releasing hormone, (d) luteinizing hormone

3 | Answer Key

1. *Mitosis:* Process to reproduce all body cells so that each cell is an exact replica of the original cell. *Meiosis:* A two-stage division process that ends with each cell having only half the number (23) of chromosomes of other body cells; process of replication for ovum and sperm only.
2. (a) 24, (b) 72
3. (a) 23, (b) 46
4. (a) XY, (b) male
5. b
6. See text, pp. 42–43
7. (a) Capacitation removes the sperm's plasma membrane and induces an attraction to the ovum. (b) Acrosomal reaction releases enzymes that break down the hyaluronic acid in the corona radiata, thereby allowing a single sperm to penetrate and fertilize the ovum.
8. a
9. c
10. d
11. e
12. b
13. (a) 7, (b) 9; Trophoblasts attach themselves to the endometrium for nourishment, the blastocyst burrows beneath the uterine lining which then thickens below the blastocyst, and the trophoblastic cells grow into the lining and form villi.
14. b
15. c
16. (a) chorion, (b) amnion
17. 350 mL at 20 weeks; after 20 weeks, amniotic fluid ranges from 700–1000 mL; the fluid is slightly alkaline and contains albumin, uric acid, creatinine, lecithin, sphingomyelin, bilirubin, vernix, leukocytes, epithelial cells, enzymes, and lanugo.
18. (a) decidua vera, (b) decidua basalis, (c) chorion, (d) amnion, (e) decidua capsularis
19. See text, pp. 46–48
20. For the process through which the placenta develops, see text, p. 48. The maternal side appears red and fleshlike and is made up of the decidua basalis and its circulation. The fetal side appears shiny and gray and consists of the chorionic villi and their circulation; the placenta at term weighs 400–600 g, and its diameter is 15–20 cm (5.9–7.9 in).
21. Answers may include: metabolic, transport, endocrine, immunologic.
22. See text, p. 22
23. The significant observations that you would want to make about the placenta would include determining the presence of all cotyledons, the presence of large infarcts or clots in the placenta, and the site of the umbilical insertion on the placenta. These observations will give you clues to potential problems for the newborn. The absence of cotyledons would indicate a need to have the clinician check the mother for retained placental fragments that could cause postpartum hemorrhage later.
24. (a) The embryonic stage starts on day 15 and continues until approximately the eighth week or until the embryo reaches a crown-rump (c-r) length of 3 cm or 1.2 inches. (b) By the end of the eighth week, every organ system and external structures are present.
25. (a) 1, (b) 2, (c) Wharton's jelly, (d) prevent compression of the umbilical cord in utero
26. oxygenated, to; deoxygenated, from
27. (a) ductus arteriosus, (b) foramen ovale, (c) inferior vena cava, (d) ductus venosus, (e) umbilical vein, (f) umbilical arteries
28. Fetal circulation differs significantly from infant and adult circulation in that the fetus's oxygenated blood originates from the placenta and flows into the right atrium. It then moves through the foramen ovale (because of the low resistance on the left side of the fetal heart) and

out the aorta to provide the head and upper body with highly oxygenated blood. Very little oxygenated blood flows into the lungs because they are collapsed and offer a high resistance to blood flow. The blood that goes through the pulmonary artery is shunted into the aorta through the ductus arteriosus, bypassing the lungs to supply the rest of the body. See text Chapter 21 for natal circulation.

29. c

30. (a) 16 weeks; (b) 13.5 cm C–R, 15 cm C–H, 200 g; (c) 20 weeks; (d) 4 weeks; (e) 16 weeks; (f) Yes, eyes close at the 10th week and then reopen about the 28th week of gestation.

31. Many factors can influence the development of the embryo or fetus. Significant factors include the quality of the sperm or ova, teratogenic agents such as drugs and radiation, and maternal nutrition. Others you might have identified are any of the complications of pregnancy, such as maternal diabetes, hypertension, or TORCH infections.

32. 8–12

33. (a) Lack of conception despite unprotected sexual intercourse for at least 12 months; (b) Difficulty in conceiving because both partners have decreased fecundity.

34. You could discuss self-care actions that can support fertility, for example: avoiding douching and artificial lubricants that alter vaginal pH and adopting positions during intercourse that support retention of sperm. For further self-care measures, see text, p. 65, Table 4–2.

35. See text, pp. 66–68

36. a

37. d

38. c

39. b

40. g

41. e

42. f

43. See text, p. 73, Table 4–4

44. (a) Induces ovulation; dosage range 50–250 mg per day orally, starting day 3 to 5 after menses; can cause hot flushes. (b) A combination of FSH and LH administered IM every day during first half of cycle to stimulate follicular development; monitor serum estradiol levels and ultrasound. (c) Used to treat hyperprolactemia; side effects may include nausea, diarrhea, dizziness, headaches. (d) Administered via continuous infusion pump; treatment period varies from 2 to 4 weeks; may require drugs to augment the various phases of reproductive cycle.

45. a

46. See text, pp. 74–76

47. A possible nursing diagnosis that would apply is Disturbance in self-esteem related to infertility. This diagnosis depends on how successful the couple is in adjusting to the loss of the ability to conceive a child. Other nursing diagnoses that might apply are Ineffective individual (or family) coping related to inability to accept infertility, or Grieving related to loss of fertility if the couple has made the decision to accept their childless status.

48. Defining characteristics that are present include: negative body image (". . . my body can't do what it should"); low self-esteem (expressed feelings of failure); failure in role performance ("I am such a failure as a woman").

49. b

50. karyotype

51. c

52. Each child has a 50% chance of developing Huntington's chorea. For diagram, see text, p. 82, Figure 4–13.

53. Because cystic fibrosis is an autosomal recessive disorder, an affected parent must have two genes for the disorder (that is, be homozygous). Thus, with one affected parent and one normal parent, none of the children would have the disorder, but all would be carriers of an abnormal gene for the disorder. See text, p. 83, Figure 4–14.

54. See text, p. 89, Figure 4–18. We hope you have learned interesting and helpful information about your family to facilitate your self-care.

55. (a) amniotic fluid, (b) basal body temperature, (c) human chorionic gonadotropin, (d) human chorionic somatomammotropin, (e) human menopausal gonadotropin, (f) human placental lactogen